GENETIC AND ENVIRONMENTAL HEARING LOSS: SYNDROMIC AND NONSYNDROMIC

BOOKS PUBLISHED BY ALAN R. LISS, INC.
FOR MARCH OF DIMES BIRTH DEFECTS FOUNDATION

Birth Defects Compendium, Second Edition, Daniel Bergsma, *Editor*

BIRTH DEFECTS: ORIGINAL ARTICLE SERIES

1980 — Volume XVI

No. 1   Enzyme Therapy in Genetic Diseases: 2, Robert J. Desnick, *Editor*
No. 2   In Vitro Epithelia and Birth Defects, B. Shannon Danes, *Editor*
No. 3   Diet in Pregnancy: A Randomized Controlled Trial of Nutritional Supplements,
         by David Rush, Zena Stein, and Mervyn Susser
No. 4   Morphogenesis and Malformation of the Ear, Robert J. Gorlin, *Editor*
No. 5   Dentistry in the Interdisciplinary Treatment of Genetic Diseases, Carlos F. Salinas
         and Ronald J. Jorgenson, *Editors*
No. 7   Genetic and Environmental Hearing Loss: Syndromic and Nonsyndromic,
         L. Stefan Levin and Connie H. Knight, *Editors*

See pages 91—92 for other volumes in this series published by Alan R. Liss, Inc.

March of Dimes Birth Defects Foundation
Birth Defects: Original Article Series, Volume XVI, Number 7, 1980

GENETIC AND ENVIRONMENTAL HEARING LOSS: SYNDROMIC AND NONSYNDROMIC

The Second Annual Symposium on Craniofacial Dysmorphology
Held in Chicago, Illinois, June 24, 1979

Sponsored by the Society of Craniofacial Genetics, The National
Academy of Gallaudet College, the March of Dimes Birth Defects
Foundation, and The Johns Hopkins School of Medicine

Editors:

L. Stefan Levin, DDS, MSD
Symposium Chairman

Connie H. Knight, MA
The National Academy of Gallaudet College

Assistant Editor:

Sue Conde Greene
March of Dimes Birth Defects Foundation

ALAN R. LISS, INC., NEW YORK

To enhance medical communication in the birth defects field,
the March of Dimes Birth Defects Foundation publishes the
Birth Defects Compendium (Second Edition), an *Original
Article Series, Syndrome Identification,* a *Reprint Series,*
and provides a series of films and related brochures.

Further information can be obtained from:

March of Dimes Birth Defects Foundation
Medical Education Division
1275 Mamaroneck Avenue
White Plains, New York 10605

Published by:

Alan R. Liss, Inc.
150 Fifth Avenue
New York, New York 10011

Library of Congress Cataloging in Publication Data

Symposium on Craniofacial Dysmorphology, 2d, Chicago,
   1979.
   Genetic and environmental hearing loss.

   (Birth defects original article series; v. 16, no. 7)
   Bibliography: p.
   Includes index.
   1. Deafness—Genetic aspects—Congresses.
2. Deafness—Etiology—Congresses.   3. Ear—Abnormalities
—Congresses. I. Levin, L. Stefan.   II. Knight,
Connie H.   III. Greene, Sue Conde.   IV. Society of
Craniofacial Genetics.   V. Title.   VI. Series.
RG626.B63   vol. 16, no. 7   [RF292]   617.8'9   80-39615
ISBN 0-8451-1040-3
Printed in the United States of America

Contents

Contributors   ix

Preface
    L. Stefan Levin and Connie H. Knight   1

Childhood Hearing Loss: Epidemiology
and Implications
    Jerome D. Schein   3

Morphogenesis and Teratogenesis of the Middle Ear
in Animals
    Tina F. Jaskoll   9

Pathogenesis of Hereditary Inner Ear Abnormalities
in Animals
    Robert J. Ruben   29

Nonsyndromic Deafness
    Walter E. Nance   35

Central Deafness: Fact or Fiction?
    Charles I. Berlin   47

Hereditary Hearing Loss and Ear Dysplasia–Renal
Adysplasia Syndromes: Syndrome Delineation
and Possible Pathogenesis
    Michael Melnick   59

Hereditary Hearing Loss Associated With
Musculoskeletal Malformations
    Robert J. Gorlin   73

Index   89

Contributors

Charles I. Berlin, PhD, Louisiana State University Medical Center, Kresge Hearing Research Laboratory, New Orleans, LA 70119 [47]

Robert J. Gorlin, DDS, MS, Department of Oral Pathology and Genetics, University of Minnesota, Minneapolis, MN 55455 [73]

Tina F. Jaskoll, PhD, Laboratory of Developmental Biology, Section of Biochemistry and Nutrition, Department of Basic Sciences, School of Dentistry—GER 319, University of Southern California, Los Angeles, CA 90007 [9]

Connie H. Knight, MA, Public Services, The National Academy of Gallaudet College, Washington, DC 20022 [1]

L. Stefan Levin, DDS, MSD, Department of Otolaryngology, The Johns Hopkins Hospital, Baltimore, MD 21205 [1]

Michael Melnick, DDS, PhD, Laboratory of Developmental Biology, Andrus Gerontology Center—325, University of Southern California, University Park, Los Angeles, CA 90007 [59]

Walter E. Nance, MD, PhD, Department of Human Genetics, Medicine and Pediatrics, Medical College of Virginia, Virginia Commonwealth University, Richmond, VA 23298 [35]

Robert J. Ruben, MD, Developmental Otobiology Laboratory, Rose F. Kennedy Center for Human Growth and Development; Department of Otorhinolaryngology, Albert Einstein College of Medicine of Yeshiva University; Montefiore Hospital and Medical Center; Bronx, New York 10461 [29]

Jerome D. Schein, PhD, Deafness Research and Training Center, New York University School of Education, New York, NY 10003 [3]

The number in brackets following each contributor's affiliation is the opening page number of that author's article.

Preface

Despite the fact that hearing impairment is one of the most prevalent chronic disabilities in the United States, the etiologic heterogeneity of this disability and the special health care needs of deaf patients too frequently go unrecognized by medical professionals. In part, this unfortunate situation exists because training programs in the health care fields typically do not deal with deafness; thus, students learn little about deafness and subsequently, as practicing clinicians, have the same misconceptions about deafness and deaf people as does the general population.

The purpose of this symposium, "Genetic and Environmental Hearing Loss: Syndromic and Nonsyndromic," was to provide insight into the etiology and pathogenesis of hearing impairment in order to educate health care professionals. To achieve this goal, a forum was provided in which investigators conducting research in hearing impairment could present their views to individuals working directly with the hearing impaired.

This symposium — which was presented at the March of Dimes Birth Defects Foundation's Birth Defects Conference in Chicago, Illinois on June 24, 1979 — was the second sponsored by the Society of Craniofacial Genetics, and was supported by the generous cosponsorship of the Gallaudet College National Academy, the March of Dimes Birth Defects Foundation, and The Johns Hopkins University School of Medicine. The first symposium of the Society, "Developmental Aspects of Craniofacial Dysmorphology," was also published as part of the Birth Defects Original Article Series (Volume XV, Number 8, 1979).

The editors thank Dr. Joe Leigh Simpson for his help during the preparation of the symposium and Ms. Terri Baker and Ms. Joanne Frantz for their secretarial assistance.

L. Stefan Levin, DDS, MSD
Connie H. Knight, MA

Birth Defects: Original Article Series, Volume XVI, Number 7, page 1
© **1980 March of Dimes Birth Defects Foundation**

Childhood Hearing Loss: Epidemiology and Implications

Jerome D. Schein, PhD

Childhood deafness presents serious obstacles to normal psychologic and social development. Hearing loss affects development because it restricts communication and thereby inhibits normal language acquisition. While their cognitive and language acquisition abilities are usually intact, hearing-impaired children do not receive sufficient auditory input to develop language from hearing the speech around them. Many variables—locus, degree, etiology, age at onset, family, and educational factors— influence the development of the hearing-impaired child.

The presence of a hearing loss need not inevitably lead to negative consequences. Given early and appropriate management, deaf children can live thoroughly satisfactory and productive lives. Counter measures, especially early educational intervention, can prevent the worst effects of childhood hearing loss. The deaf child can become a literate deaf adult, contributing economically and socially to the community, and enjoying full citizenship.

The many variables of childhood deafness have made it difficult to define, and epidemiologic study has been hindered by lack of a clear definition. Carefully designed epidemiologic studies of childhood hearing loss can be a valuable tool in research, in identification, and in the management and planning of services for deaf people. This paper will review two major epidemiologic studies of childhood hearing loss and suggest directions for future investigations.

Birth Defects: Original Article Series, Volume XVI, Number 7, pages 3—7
© **1980 March of Dimes Birth Defects Foundation**

EXISTING EPIDEMIOLOGIC STUDIES

Two major epidemiologic investigations of childhood hearing loss have been undertaken—the Annual Survey of Hearing Impaired Children and Youth (ASHICY) [1] and the National Census of the Deaf Population (NCDP) [2]. Below are major findings concerning prevalence, geographic distribution, sex, and race. Also included are etiologic findings of leading geneticists studying deafness.

Gross Prevalence Rates.   Table 1 shows the estimated number of hearing-impaired persons, based on self reports [2]. A hearing-impaired person is one who answers yes to the question, "Do you have any trouble hearing in one or both ears?" A deaf person is one who reports he cannot hear and understand speech. Audiometric surveys produce larger estimates of the total number of hearing-impaired persons. The reason for this disparity is that, in general, people tend not to report increases in hearing thresholds for speech until they reach 30–35 dB, whereas most audiometric surveys consider deviations at or above 20 dB as impairments.

The prevalence rates in Table 1 show that the estimates are much larger than those previously considered. Deafness, without regard to age at onset, occurs at a rate of 837/100,000. For those born deaf or deafened before 19 years of age, the prevalence rate is more than double the previous estimate of 1/1,000. The 1/1,000 rate applies

Table 1. Prevalence and Prevalence Rates for Hearing Impairments in the Civilian Noninstitutionalized Population, by Degree and Age at Onset: United States, 1971.

Degree	Age at Onset	Number	Rate per 100,000
All hearing impairment	All ages	13,362,842	6,603
Significant bilateral	All ages	6,548,842	3,236
Deafness	All ages	1,767,046	873
	Prevocational[a]	410,522	203
	Prelingual[b]	201,626	100

[a]Prior to 19 years of age.
[b]Prior to 3 years of age.

only to those who report losing their hearing before 3 years of age, the so-called prelingually deaf group. Clearly, how one chooses to define "childhood" will greatly affect estimates of the prevalence of childhood deafness. Classifications based on degree of impairment also affect statistics.

Geographic Distribution. The prevalence rates in Table 2 show the great difference in rates for hearing impairment and deafness by regions of the United States [2]. Though these are not incidence rates, they do suggest the value of local studies to isolate causal factors.

Since these figures are from the NCPD, where methods of data collection and the definitions used in classification are the same for each region, results from the regions can be directly compared. The general trend of lowest prevalence rates in the northeast region and highest ones in the north central region has appeared consistently in US

Table 2. Distribution of Hearing-Impaired Population by Regions: United States, 1971.

United States and Regions[a]	Hearing Impaired	Deaf	Prevocationally Deaf
United States	13,362,842	1,767,046	410,522
Northeast	2,891,380	337,022	83,909
North Central	3,683,226	541,465	135,653
South	4,280,177	562,756	123,260
West	2,508,059	325,803	67,700
Rate per 100,000 Population			
United States	6,603	873	203
Northeast	5,977	697	173
North Central	6,563	965	242
South	6,807	895	196
West	7,170	931	194

[a]Northeast: Connecticut, Maine, Massachusetts, New Hampshire, New Jersey, New York, Pennsylvania, Rhode Island, Vermont
North Central: Illinois, Indiana, Iowa, Kansas, Michigan, Minnesota, Missouri, Nebraska, North Dakota, Ohio, South Dakota, Wisconsin
South: Alabama, Arkansas, Delaware, District of Columbia, Florida, Georgia, Kentucky, Louisiana, Maryland, Mississippi, North Carolina, Oklahoma, South Carolina, Tennessee, Texas, Virginia, West Virginia
West: Alaska, Arizona, California, Colorado, Hawaii, Idaho, Montana, Nevada, New Mexico, Oregon, Utah, Washington, Wyoming

data. The common explanations are that 1) areas around seaports tend to be wealthier than inland areas; hence, medical care, diet, and similar conditions are better, 2) climate is milder on the seacoast, 3) iodine deficiency is less common, and 4) consanguinity is lower than in more isolated areas. All of these factors affect hearing impairment.

Sex and Race. ASHICY finds that over the years distribution between the sexes has remained nearly constant. For the 44,000 students in the ASHICY sample, there are about 118 males for every 100 females. This male preference appears routinely in studies of deaf populations.

With respect to race, the NCDP and ASHICY figures differ. NCDP found lower rates for deafness among nonwhites. ASHICY found nonwhites represented in their sample in about the same proportions as they occur in the total population. The NCDP suspected that its findings reflect economic, not epidemiologic, factors.

Etiology. Extensive research by Nance, Fraser, and others suggests that genetic factors are more frequently responsible for deafness than had previously been suspected. The most striking finding for Fraser, as he reviewed his etiologic investigation of 3,500 cases of profound childhood deafness, was "the pronounced *heterogeneity* of biological causation involving an entity which, from the educational, social, and even medical, point of view, is often regarded as relatively homogeneous" [3].

FUTURE DIRECTIONS

Research in the epidemiology of childhood hearing impairment has been hindered in the past by lack of agreement in the health fields on the major parameters defining the condition. This lack of a clear definition has been confusing, for obviously the way in which the population is delimited influences findings.

At this stage in the epidemiologic art, it may be appropriate to consider more carefully the implications of childhood hearing loss, based on clinical experience and the results of demographic and psychologic research, in order to develop definitions that reflect functional effects. With an awareness of the implications of childhood hearing impairment of different degrees, ages at onset, etiologies, and perhaps other factors, researchers may be better able to study the entire hearing-impaired population and discriminate accurately among subgroups. Thus, the variety of characteristics of the early hearing-impaired population need not continue to be a confusing factor, but rather can be used to clarify differential effects of the various parameters.

Carefully designed epidemiologic studies of childhood hearing impairment will be a valuable tool in medical and educational management. Data leading to identifying etiologies can, as with rubella, lead to the reduction or eradication of certain etiologies and to refining methods of identifying affected individuals through high-risk categorizations. Information about behavioral characteristics of hearing-impaired infants and children can be used in developing successful intervention programs. An accurate picture of the demographic composition, including geographic distribution of the hearing-impaired population can be used in planning and implementing services for deaf people.

REFERENCES

1. Ries PW, Bateman DL, Schildroth A: "Ethnic Background in Relation to Other Characteristics of Hearing Impaired Students in the United States." Series D, No. 15. Washington, DC: Gallaudet College, Office of Demographic Studies, 1975.
2. Schein JD, Delk MT: "The Deaf Population of the United States." Silver Springs, MD: National Association of the Deaf, 1974.
3. Fraser GR: "The Causes of Profound Deafness in Childhood." Baltimore: The Johns Hopkins University Press, 1976, p 348.

Morphogenesis and Teratogenesis of the Middle Ear in Animals*

Tina F. Jaskoll, PhD

Congenital malformations of the ear occur in 1 of 3,800 live births [1]. Only a small percentage of live newborns has major abnormalities of the middle ear. However, middle ear abnormalities are frequently found in a variety of syndromes, eg the Treacher Collins syndrome [2, 3], 1st and 2nd branchial arch dysplasia (hemifacial microsomia) [2, 3], and in patients exposed to disease and medication in intrauterine life [2, 3]. Human middle ear studies have emphasized the diagnosis [4–6], classification [1, 3], and treatment of malformations [4–6]. Morphologic studies of the development of the human middle ear are available [7–9], but little is known about the developmental dynamics of this region. A comprehensive understanding of middle ear development would provide insight into the etiology and pathogenesis of congenital middle ear malformations.

The middle ear region, with structures derived from all 3 germ layers, as well as the neural crest, is a complex, yet intriguing system. Since the human middle ear is relatively inaccessible, one must rely on the study of animal models. Because the objective of animal studies is a better understanding of human development, it would be best to conduct studies in mammalian systems; however, maternal physiology, maternal resorption of the fetus, and fetal inaccessibility for experimental manipulation in these systems often hinder investigations. Therefore, other animal models, such as the chick embryo, are used extensively.

*Supported by NIH grants CA-18622 and NS-13924 and by NIDR-NIH grants DE 02848 and DE 07006.

Birth Defects: Original Article Series, Volume XVI, Number 7, pages 9–28
© 1980 March of Dimes Birth Defects Foundation

This paper will briefly describe normal middle ear development and development of the fenestra ovalis region in animal models and will present the results of teratogen studies. The possible etiology of middle ear anomalies will also be discussed.

THE DEVELOPMENTAL ANATOMY OF THE MIDDLE EAR

The mammalian middle ear consists of a chain of 3 ossicles—the malleus, incus, and stapes—which transmit sound from the tympanic membrane to the fenestra ovalis (oval window). Figure 1 illustrates an idealized cross section of the middle ear of a 9-day-old mouse; the ossicles are not yet suspended within the middle ear cavity. The stapedial footplate inserts into the fenestra ovalis, the boundary between the middle and inner ear. The trilaminar tympanic membrane is the boundary between the middle and external ears. The inner aspect of the membrane is continuous with the endodermal epithelium of the tympanic cavity, its outer aspect is continuous with the ectodermal epithelium of the external auditory meatus, and the intermediate lamina propria consists of densely packed connective tissue.

The development of the mammalian middle ear is intimately associated with that of the external ear, mandible, and maxilla. The malleus and incus, as well as the mandible and maxilla, are derived from the 1st (mandibular) branchial arch [7–9]. Based on morphologic studies by Anson, Hanson, and co-workers [7–9], the long arm of the incus and the malleus manubrium are probably derived from the 2nd (hyoid) branchial arch. The 2nd branchial arch also contributes to formation of the stapes. Extirpation studies [10, 11], histochemical studies [12, 13], and morphologic studies [7, 8, 14, 15] demonstrate that the stapedial footplate receives contributions from both the otic capsule and the 2nd branchial arch. The middle ear cavity develops as an expansion of the lateral portion of the 1st pharyngeal (branchial) pouch (tubotympanic sulcus); the 1st branchial cleft forms the external auditory meatus. The epithelium of the tympanic membrane is derived from the epithelium of the 1st pouch and

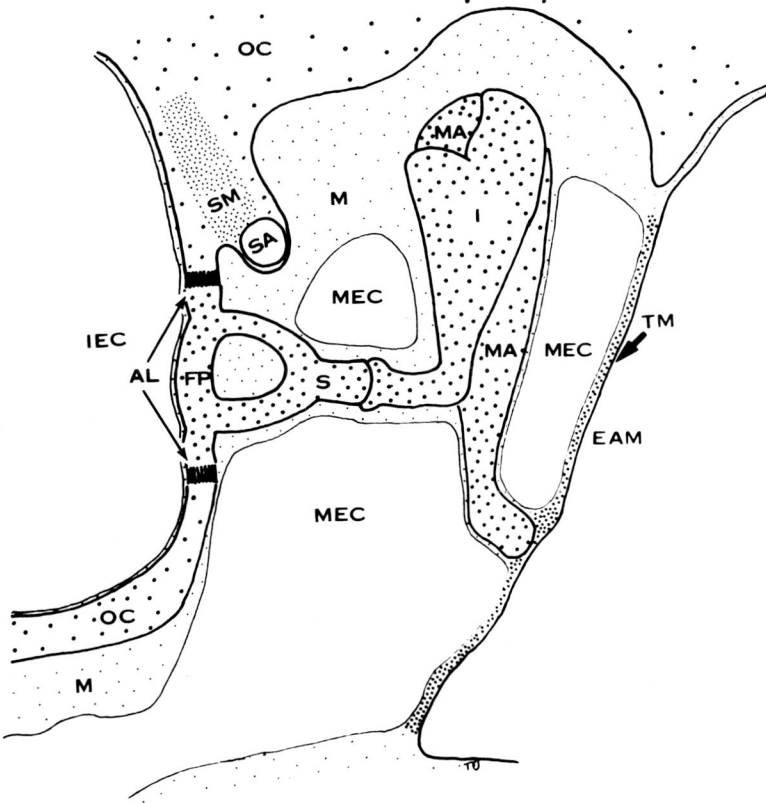

Fig. 1. An idealized cross section through the middle ear of a 9-day-old mouse. The malleus, incus, and stapes span the space from the tympanic membrane to the fenestra ovalis. The stapedial footplate is suspended within the fenestra ovalis by the annular ligament. The middle ear cavity does not completely surround the ossicles; the body of the incus is surrounded by undifferentiated mesenchyme. The stapedial artery persists in the rodent although it disappears during human development. (From Jaskoll [15].) Key: AL—annular ligament, EAM—external auditory meatus, FP—stapedial footplate, I—incus, IEC—inner ear cavity, M—undifferentiated mesenchyme, MA—malleus, MEC—middle ear cavity, OC—otic capsule, S—stapes, SA—stapedial artery, SM—stapedius muscle, TM—tympanic membrane.

cleft. The pinna is derived from both the 1st and 2nd arches.

Abnormal development of the 1st and 2nd branchial arches may therefore result in anomalies of any or all the following structures: maxilla, mandible, external ear, and auditory ossicles. Since the long arm of the incus and the malleus manubrium are derived from the 2nd branchial arch, malformations of these structures are frequently associated with malformations of the stapes [5, 6]. A thorough knowledge of middle ear development of animal models [14–19] and its relevance to human development is necessary prior to conducting experimental investigations on the middle ear (Table 1).

MOUSE MIDDLE EAR (TABLE 1)

The first indication of the mouse middle ear occurs 11 days post coitum when mesenchymal condensations are observed lateral to the otic capsule. By day 12, the precartilaginous condensations are recognized as the malleus, incus, and stapes. The stapedial condensation is adjacent to but not continuous with the otic capsule as seen in the 13-day fetus (Fig. 2A). The developing ossicles are embedded within undifferentiated mesenchyme. The 1st pharyngeal pouch projects laterally toward the ossicles, and its proximal and distal portions differentiate

Table 1. Comparison of Middle Ear Development

	Chick (HH stages/days)	Mouse (days gestation)	Human (weeks)
Ossicle(s) condensation	25/5	11	4–5
Ossicle(s) chondrification	32–34/7½–8	14	8
Ossicle(s) ossification			
malleus and incus	–	24/4 days postnate	16–16½
stapes	41/15	25/5 days postnate	18
Fenestra ovalis formation			
stapedial footplate fusion			
with otic capsule	32–34/7½–8	15	9–10
footplate suspended by			
annular ligament cells	35/9	15–16	10–13
annular ligament	38/12	18–22	20+
Middle ear cavity (MEC) formation			
tubotympanic sulcus formation	22–23/4	12	4
MEC surrounds ossicle(s)	38/12	36/16 days postnate	24–27
Tympanic membrane formation			
external auditory meatus	26/5	12	8
presumptive tympanic membrane	29–34/6–8	15	10
meatal plate resorption	–	23/3 days postnate	12

into the eustachian tube and middle ear cavity, respectively. The 1st branchial cleft, the presumptive external auditory meatus, is only a depression of the head epithelium at this stage of development. Chondrification of the ossicles begins on day 14. By day 16, the stapedial footplate becomes suspended in the presumptive fenestra ovalis by presumptive annular ligament cells (Fig. 2B). The middle ear region is still filled with undifferentiated mesenchyme and the middle ear cavity is located ventral to the malleus. The external auditory meatus is growing anteroventromedially as a meatal plate.

Unlike the avian and human middle ear, the middle ear of the mouse is not fully differentiated at birth (Fig. 2C). The stapedial footplate of this 2-day-old mouse is suspended by the differentiated annular ligament in the fenestra ovalis (Fig. 2C). The malleus manubrium inserts into the inner aspect of the presumptive tympanic membrane. The malleus, incus, and stapes are surrounded by loosely packed mesenchyme. Ossicle ossification begins on the 4th day after birth (Table 1); the cells adjacent to the annular ligament and ossicle joints remain cartilaginous. In the 7-day-old mouse, further development of the middle ear is observed (Fig. 2D). The stapes and incus are ossifying and the incudostapedial joint has differentiated. The endodermal epithelium of the middle ear cavity continues to expand dorsad toward the ossicles. In the mouse, the ossicles are not completely suspended within the middle ear cavity until 16 days after birth. Expansion of the tympanic cavity and associated mesenchymal elimination from the middle ear have been previously discussed [15].

Avian Middle Ear (Table 1)

The avian middle ear consists of a single ossicle, the stapes (columella), which is derived from the 2nd branchial arch [10, 11]. The stapedial condensation, first observed at Hamburger Hamilton (H.H.) [20] stages 25–27 (5 days), is initially separated from the otic capsule. By H.H. stage 32 (7½ days) the stapes is continuous with the capsule; these structures begin to ossify at H.H. stage

32–34 (7½–8 days). In the middle ear of an embryo at
H.H. stage 34 (8 days), the stapes and otic capsule are
continuous (Fig. 3A). The presumptive annular ligament
cells are chondrified. These chondrified cells dedifferen-
tiate and redifferentiate into the annular ligament (H.H.
stage 36/10 days). The differentiated middle ear at H.H.

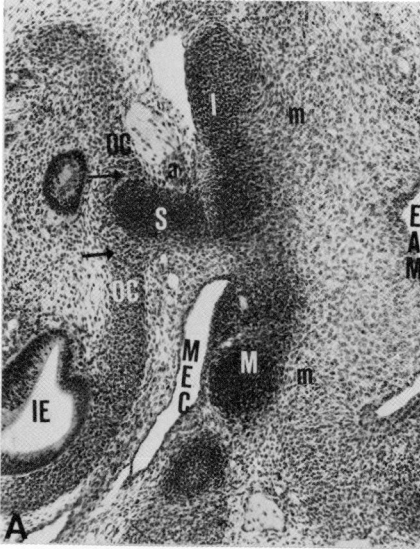

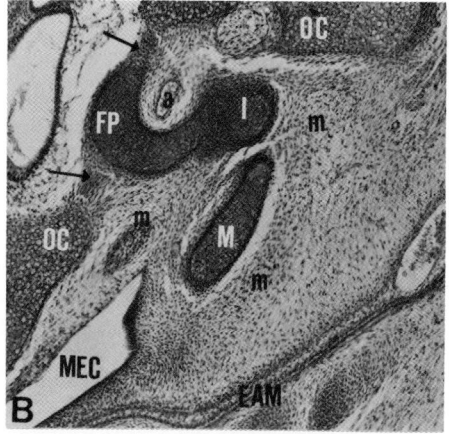

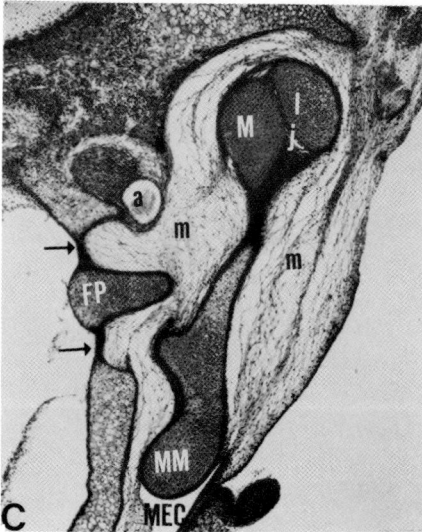

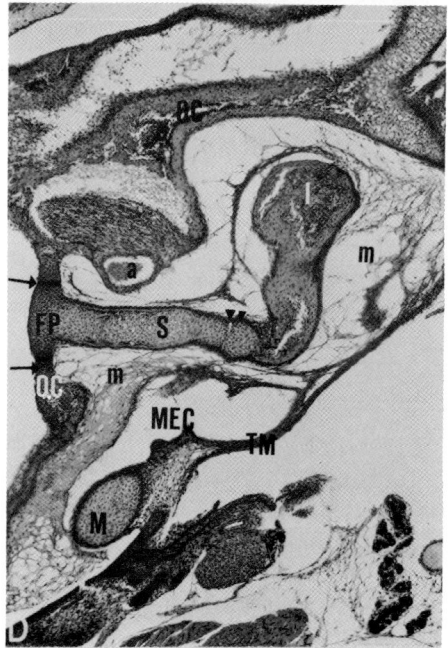

stage 38 (12 days) is seen in Figure 3B. The stapes is suspended within a middle ear cavity and inserts via the extrastapes onto the tympanic membrane. The stapedial footplate is suspended in the fenestra ovalis by the annular ligament. Details of avian middle ear development have been published elsewhere and will not be discussed here [14].

DEVELOPMENT OF THE FENESTRA OVALIS

The differentiation of human, murine, and avian middle ear structures is similar (Table 1). The simplicity of the avian middle ear with its single ossicle permits a schematic representation of the major steps in the development of the stapedial footplate and annular ligament (Fig. 4): this pattern of development of the fenestra ovalis region is analogous to that observed in mammals [15]. The stapedial (2nd branchial arch) condensation is initially separated from the otic capsule by a region of undifferentiated mesenchyme (Figs. 4A and B). The stapedial primordium moves closer to (Fig. 4C) and becomes continous with the otic capsule to form the stapedial foot-

Fig. 2. The development of the CBA/J mouse middle ear. A) A cross section of the 13-day mouse fetus. The prechondroblasts of the stapes, incus, and malleus are more densely packed than those of the otic capsule. The stapedial footplate is continuous with the otic capsule, although the 2 cell populations are distinct (arrows). The ossicles are embedded within undifferentiated mesenchyme ($\times$ 160). B) In the 16-day fetus, the stapedial footplate is suspended with the fenestra ovalis by the presumptive annular ligament cells (arrows). The chondrifying ossicles are surrounded by undifferentiated mesenchyme. The external auditory meatus has invaginated anteroventromedially as a meatal plate ($\times$ 160). C) In the 2-day-old mouse, the footplate is suspended in the fenestra ovalis by the differentiated annular ligament (arrows). The incudomalleolar joint is beginning to differentiate. The malleus manubrium inserts into the endodermal epithelium of the middle ear cavity. The external auditory meatus is ventral to the middle ear cavity ($\times$ 100). D) In the 7-day-old mouse the stapes and incus are ossifying. The incudostapedial joint (double arrows) has differentiated; the tissue adjacent to the joint remains cartilaginous. The middle ear cavity is expanding around the ossicles, but at this stage the stapes, incus, and head of the malleus are still surrounded by undifferentiated mesenchyme ($\times$ 100). Key: a—stapedial artery, EAM—external auditory meatus, FP—stapedial footplate, I—incus, IE—inner ear, j—incudomalleolar joint, m—undifferentiated mesenchyme, M—malleus, MM—malleus manubrium, MEC—middle ear cavity, OC—otic capsule, S—stapes, TM—tympanic membrane.

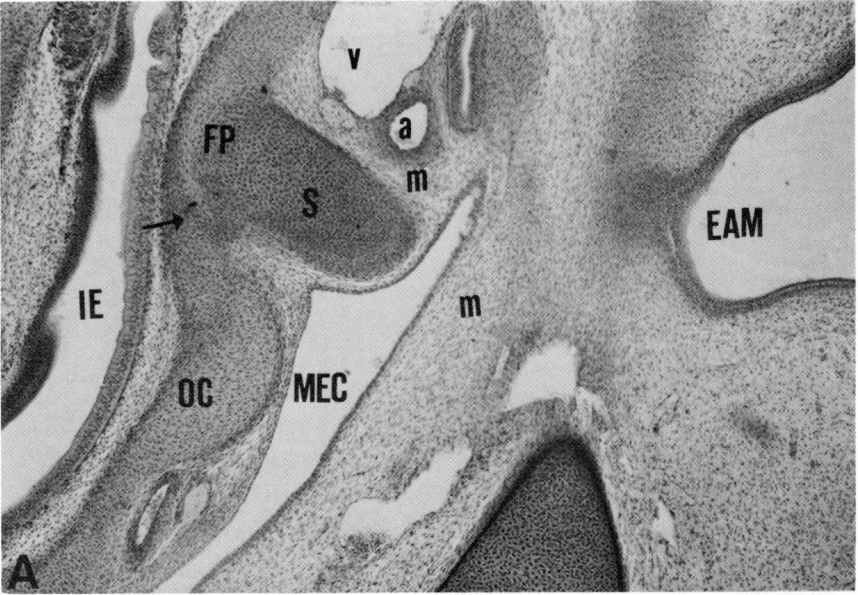

A

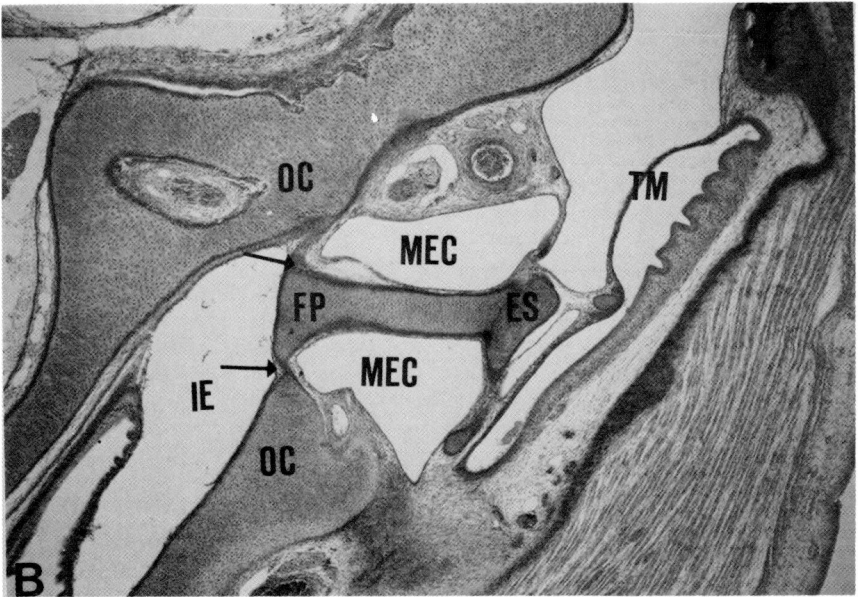

B

plate (Fig. 4D). All of the cells within the fenestra ovalis region are potentially chondrogenic based on histochemical evidence [15]. The presumptive annular ligament at the footplate-capsule interface is distinguished from the chondrocytes of the stapedial footplate and proximal otic capsule by staining characteristics (Fig. 4D). These presumptive ligamental cells lose their chondrogenic potential and differentiate into the annular ligament, which suspends the stapedial footplate in the fenestra ovalis (Figs. 4E and F); this event is probably under the influence of the stapedial footplate and proximal otic capsule [14].

TERATOGEN INVESTIGATIONS

Teratogens have been used to disrupt morphogenesis and produce embryonic abnormalities [21, 22]. Craniofacial anomalies have been observed after teratogen treatment; the type and frequency of these abnormalities depend as much on the time of administration as on tissue sensitivity [21, 22]. The administration of teratogens with different mechanisms (eg antimitotic agents and agents which impede morphogenetic movements) at the same embryonic stage and subsequent analysis of their effects on the embryo might permit determination of the specific developmental events which are disrupted [22]. However, identical structural defects may be the result of different pathogenetic events, as teratogens could activate one or more mechanisms as well as a chain reaction of responses to a particular initiating mechanism [22].

Teratogenic investigations have been conducted on the middle ear region (Table 2). Morphologic descriptions of

---

Fig. 3.   The development of the chick middle ear. A) In the HH stage 34 (8 days) the chondrified stapes and otic capsule are continuous. The region of the presumptive annular ligament (arrow) is also chondrified (compare with Figs. 2A and B). The middle ear cavity is ventral to the ossicle. B) The differentiated middle ear is seen at HH stage 38 (12 days). The footplate is suspended in the fenestra ovalis by the ligament (arrow). The stapes, inserting onto the tympanic membrane by the extrastapes (ES), is suspended within a middle ear cavity ($\times$ 63). Key: a—stapedial artery, EAM—external auditory meatus, ES—extrastapes, FP—stapedial footplate, IE—inner ear, m—undifferentiated mesenchyme, MEC—middle ear cavity, OC—otic capsule, S—stapes, TM—tympanic membrane, v—vein.

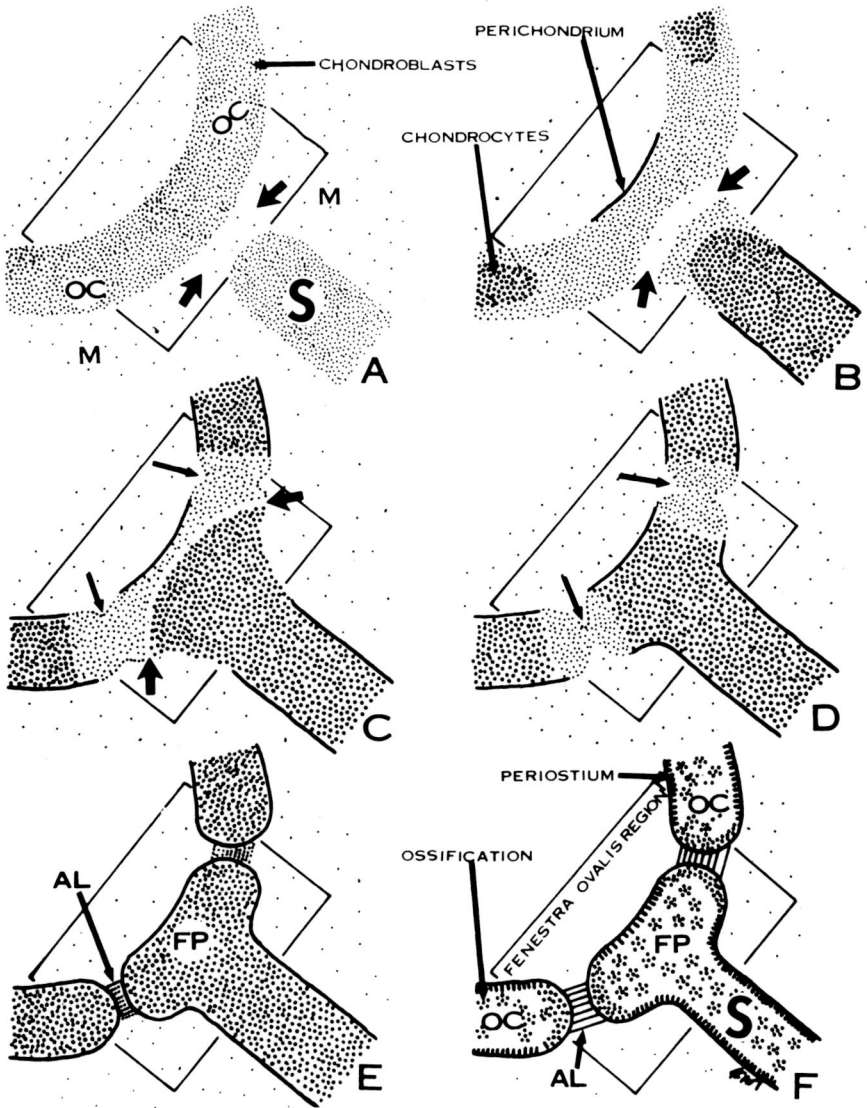

Fig. 4. Schematic drawings depicting the differentiation of the tissues of the region of the fenestra ovalis. The drawings are not to scale. A) The chondroblasts of the stapes are separated from those of the otic capsule by undifferentiated mesenchyme (arrows). B) The cell population of the stapes and otic capsule are closer together but still separated by undifferentiated mesenchyme (arrows). C) The stapes and otic capsule are continuous (heavy arrows). The cells are distinguishable from the adjacent skeletal elements by staining characteristics. D) The stapes and capsule consist almost entirely of chondrocytes and

Table 2. The Effect of Teratogens on Middle Ear

Drug	Animal	Abnormality	Reference
Vitamin A	Mouse	Ossicles, MEC, TM	[31]
	Rat	Ossicles, MEC, TM	[23, 28]
	Hamster	Ossicles, MEC, TM	[26]
Triazene	Mouse	Ossicles, MEC, TM	[24, 25]
Thalidomide	Monkey	Ossicles (less severe), MEC	[24, 25]
5-Fluoro-2-desoxyuridine	Rat	Ossicles, MEC	[27]
5-Fluorouracil	Chick	Ossicle, MEC, TM	[15]
Triethylenemelamine	Chick	Ossicle, MEC, TM	[15]
Hadacidin	Chick	Ossicle, MEC, TM	[33]
	Hamster	None	[32]
β-2-Thienylalanine	Chick	None	[15]
β-Aminoproprionitrile	Rat	Ectopic cartilages	[29]
	Chick	Ossicle (rare)	[15]
Triamcinolone	Mouse	None	[31]
Dexamethasone	Mouse	None	[31]
Trypan blue	Rat	Ossicles, MEC	[30]
Pilocarpine	Chick	Ossicle	[15]

middle ear structures are presented in only a few of the studies [15, 23–25]. More frequently, however, the middle ear is simply described as abnormal, rudimentary, or absent [26–28]. Detailed studies of the effects of teratogens on the avian and murine middle ear have been presented elsewhere [15, 31]; a summary of the results will be presented here.

Teratogens which induce anomalies of 1st and 2nd branchial arch derivatives [21, 34] were selected. These teratogens were administered to the avian embryo over a wide range of developmental stages and recovered at

are nearly completely surrounded by a perichondrium. At the stapedial foot-plate-otic capsule interface, chondroblast populations are still visible, and the cells at the isthmus represent the presumptive annular ligament (arrows). E) The footplate is suspended within the fenestra ovalis by the annular ligament. F) The differentiation of the annular ligament is now complete, and collagen fibers are visible therein. (From Jaskoll TF and Maderson PFA: A histological study of the development of the avian middle ear and tympanum. Anat Rec 190:177–200, 1978, with permission.) Key: AL—annular ligament, FP—stapedial footplate, M—undifferentiated mesenchyme, OC—otic capsule, S—stapes.

H.H. stages 35–36 (8–9 days) [15, 31]. Vitamin A and
glucocorticosteroid analogs were administered to pregnant mice on day 8 or 9 of pregnancy (plug equals day 0)
and recovered at day 17. All fetuses were staged under
the dissecting microscope, examined for gross abnormalities, and evaluated histologically [15].

Three types of ossicular abnormalities were observed
in these studies [15, 33]. In the Type I abnormality, the
stapedial footplate was continuous with the otic capsule,
as illustrated in a vitamin A treated mouse (Fig. 5A) and
a triethylenemelamine (TEM) treated chick (Fig. 5B). The
annular ligament and fenestra ovalis were absent. The
area which normally differentiates into the annular ligament was chondrified and morphologically identical to the
adjacent otic capsule and footplate (Fig. 5B). The otic
tissue was enclosed in a contiguous perichondrium. In the
Type II abnormality, the stapes was separated from the
otic capsule; the stapes and otic capsule were surrounded
by separate perichondria (Fig. 6). The stapedial footplate,
annular ligament, and fenestra ovalis were absent. The
Type II abnormality was demonstrated in an untreated
mouse (Fig. 6A) and a hadacidin-treated chick (Fig. 6B).
In the Type III abnormality, the ossicles were structurally
abnormal, one or more ossicular components were absent, or the ossicles were completely absent (Fig. 5A).
The Type III abnormality was frequently associated with
stapedial footplate abnormalities found in Types I and II.
Teratogens often resulted in a combination of abnormalities. Administration of Vitamin A to pregnant mice resulted in fetuses with a fused footplate (Type I) and absent
malleus and incus (Type III) (Fig. 5A). Figure 7 summarizes the ossicular abnormalities and their associated teratogens. It is probable that other teratogens not included
in this summary also induce these middle ear defects; the
absence of morphologic descriptions in other investigations [26–30] prevents the classification of these teratogens. The middle ear was normal after glucocorticosteroid and β-2-thienylalanine treatment [15, 31].

Using many of the teratogenic agents cited in Table 2,
such as vitamin A and hadacidin, abnormalities of other

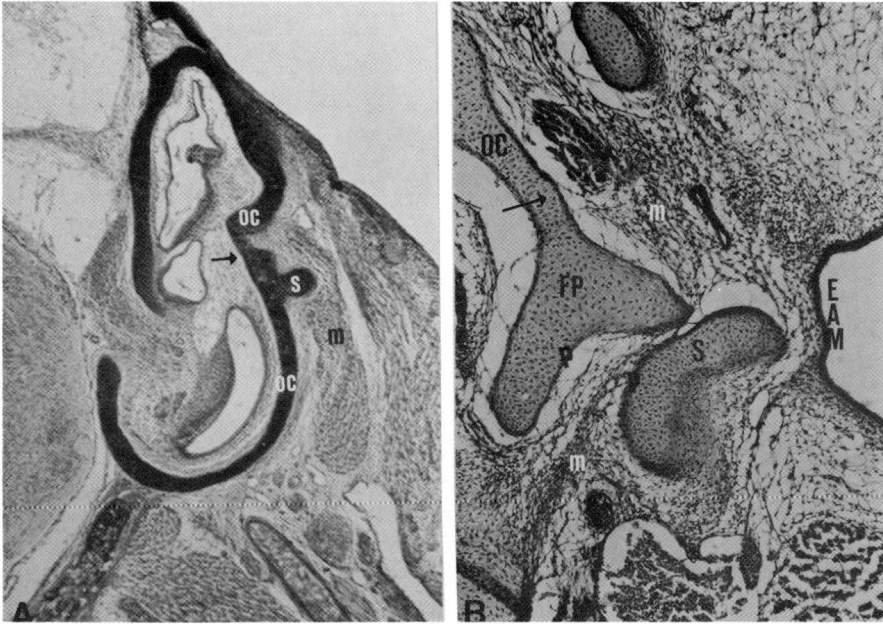

Fig. 5. A) Type I ossicle abnormality in a vitamin A treated mouse. The malleus and incus are absent ($\times$ 100). B) Triethylenemelamine (TEM) treated chick ($\times$ 120). The footplate is fused with the otic capsule. The arrow indicates the region normally occupied by the annular ligament. Note the absence of the middle ear cavity and the more densely packed mesenchyme in both animals. Key: EAM—external auditory meatus, FP—stapedial footplate, m—undifferentiated mesenchyme, OC—otic capsule, p—perichondrium, S—stapes.

middle ear components were observed. For example, the middle ear cavity was decreased in size or absent (Figs. 5 and 6) and the mesenchyme surrounding the ossicles was denser than normal (Figs. 2, 3, 5, and 6). The decreased size or absence of the middle ear cavity resulted in tympanic membrane abnormalities. Details of the effect of teratogens on other components of the middle ear have been published elsewhere and will not be discussed here [15, 33].

Anomalies of the middle ear are always associated with craniofacial abnormalities [15, 33]. Poswillo [24, 25] produced a mouse model of 1st and 2nd branchial arch dysplasia (hemifacial microsomia) by treating mice with

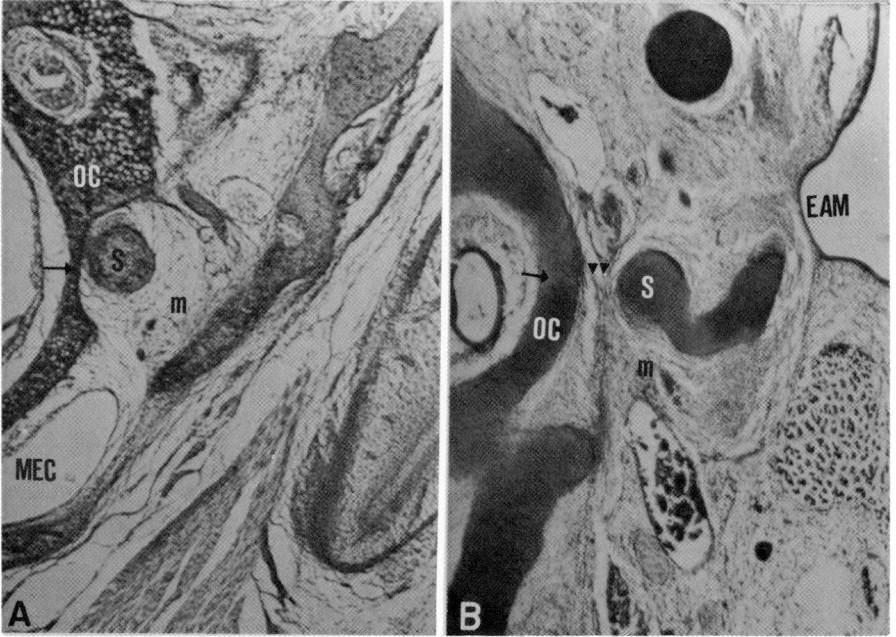

Fig. 6. A) Nonteratogen-induced Type II ossicle abnormality in 17-day mouse fetus (× 100). B) Hadacidin-treated chick (× 100). The arrow indicates the region normally occupied by the footplate. The double arrows indicate the distance between the otic capsule and stapes. Note the absence of the middle ear cavity in both animals. Key: EAM—external auditory meatus, m—undifferentiated mesenchyme, MEC—middle ear cavity, OC—otic capsule, S—stapes.

triazene. The middle ear defects in these animals were attributed to hemorrhage of the stapedial artery in the middle ear region. On the other hand, the inner ears of these animals were normal. Poswillo concluded that the inner ear was protected from the harmful effects of the hemorrhage by the otic capsule. Results of our studies [31], however, indicated that the inner ear was not always normal after treatment with teratogenic agents. Hemorrhage was seen in the inner ear, middle ear, and brain of a triamcinolone-hexacetonide-treated mouse (Fig. 8). The inner ear was abnormal and the annular ligament torn; all other middle ear structures were normal. The inner ear of this animal was not protected from the destructive effect of hemorrhage.

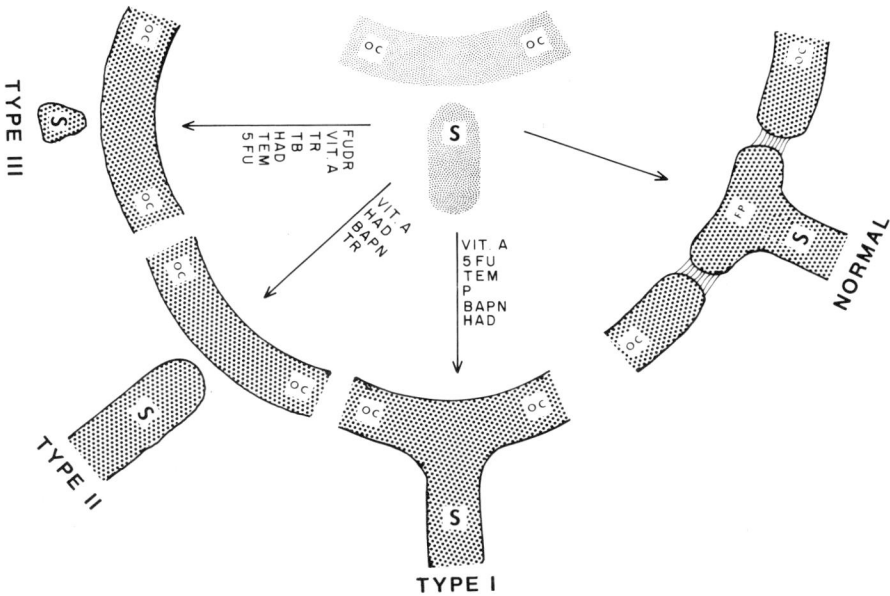

Fig. 7. A summary of the effect of teratogens on ossicle development. A normal ossicle can develop after all of the teratogens. Key: BAPN—β-amino-proprionitrile; 5 FU—5 fluorouracil; FUDR—5-fluoro-2-desoxyuridine; HAD—hadacidin; p—pilocarpine; TB—trypan blue; TEM—triethylenemelamine; TR—triazene; VIT.A—Vitamin A; FP—stapedial footplate; OC—otic capsule; S—stapes.

DISCUSSION

Morphogenesis of the middle ear ossicles can be divided into 3 events: the establishment of ossicular primordia; the differentiation of the fenestra ovalis; and the chondrification, ossification, and remodeling of the ossicles. In the early embryo, neural crest cells migrate from the mesencephalic and rhombencephalic regions into the 1st and 2nd branchial arches [35, 36]. These neural crest-derived ectomesenchymal cells proliferate to form the majority of the mesenchymal cells in the branchial arches and become the presumptive ossicles [36]. The development of the fenestra ovalis region involves 2 major steps: stapedial footplate formation and annular ligament differ-

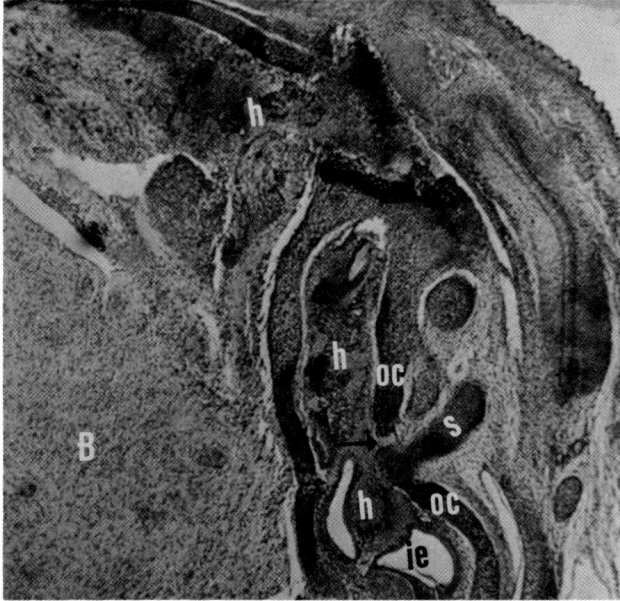

Fig. 8.   A cross section of a triamcinolone-hexacetonide-treated mouse. A hemorrhage is located within the inner ear, middle ear, and brain. The annular ligament is torn; all other middle ear structures are normal (× 63). Key: B—brain, h—hemorrhage, ie—inner ear, oc—otic capsule, s—stapes.

entiation. The stapedial primordia, composed of 2nd branchial arch ectomesenchyme, is initially separated from the otic capsule and becomes continuous with the capsule to form the stapedial footplate. The presumptive annular ligament cells at the footplate-capsule interface lose their chondrogenic potential and differentiate into the annular ligament, thereby suspending the footplate in the fenestra ovalis. During subsequent development, chondrification, ossification, and remodeling of the ossicles occur.

Structural defects of the middle ear ossicles observed in the teratogen studies (Fig. 7) could be interpreted according to this sequence of ossicular development. Complete absence of the middle ear ossicles in animal models is rare. However, malformations or absence of one or more components of the ossicles are frequently observed [15, 31, 33]; these defects are probably due to disruption of normal patterns of cell migration, proliferation, and cellular interaction in the middle ear. For example, interruption of neural crest cell migration into the branchial arches and interference in the process of cell proliferation could result in a decreased number of ectomesenchymal cells in the middle ear region. In this case, the mesenchymal primordia of the ossicles would be absent or diminished in size, leading to the absence of ossicle(s) or abnormalities of ossicular components, respectively (Type III abnormality), and the misalignment and discontinuity of the stapedial primordium and the otic capsule. Under these conditions, the stapedial shaft would remain separate from the otic capsule resulting in a Type II abnormality. Teratogen interference after stapedial footplate formation might disrupt the interactions necessary for annular ligament differentiation. The presumptive ligamental cells under these conditions would express their chondrogenic phenotype and fusion of the footplate and otic capsule would ensue (Type I abnormality).

Many of the teratogens cited have been shown to disrupt neural crest cell migration and proliferation. Morriss [37] injected excess vitamin A into pregnant rats and observed facial, otic, and brain abnormalities. In vitro experiments [37] indicated that neural crest cell migration was abnormal in the presence of vitamin A. Hassell et al [38] have conducted similar in vitro experiments on chick embryos and observed that vitamin A prevented the appearance of neural crest cells in the 1st branchial arch. Other teratogens could also interfere with neural crest cell migrations [15].

Decreased neural crest cell number could also be the result of disruption of mitosis. Many teratogens (eg hadacidin, 5-fluorouracil, and triethylenemelamine) are antimitotic agents. These drugs interfere with cell proliferation, and at higher concentrations, produce cell death, resulting in decreased numbers of crest cells in the branchial arches and malformations of the middle ear ossicles.

Middle ear abnormalities could be the result of pathogenetic events different from those discussed above. For example, skeletal development is responsive to environmental (epigenetic) factors [39]. Extirpation of optic, otic, and cranial primordia in the avian [40, 41] and amphibian [42, 43] embryos result in cranial defects. These structural defects are probably the result of abnormal stress on the developing skeleton. The results of in vitro investigations of the otic region support the importance of the environment on ossicle development [15, 44–46]. Chick and mouse otic regions were grown on the chick chorioallantoic membrane [15, 44] or in organ culture [45, 46]; the fenestra ovalis region and ossicles were abnormal. These defects were probably due to the disruption of normal cranial integrity rather than disruption of cell migration or proliferation. We are currently investigating the role of environmental factors on cranial development using the technique of long-term cultivation of chick embryos in vitro to determine the importance of extrinsic biomechanical factors in middle ear development [31].

It is obvious that our ignorance of middle ear development far exceeds our knowledge. Further investigations into the etiology and pathogenesis of middle ear anomalies in animal models should be conducted to answer many of the still outstanding questions.

ACKNOWLEDGMENTS

The author thanks Drs. M. Melnick, H.C. Slavkin, and P.F.A. Maderson for their support and advice.

REFERENCES

1. Lapayowker MS: Congenital anomalies of the middle ear. Radiologic Clinics of North America 12:463–471, 1974.
2. Gorlin RJ, Pindborg JJ, Cohen MM Jr: "Syndromes of the Head and Neck." New York:McGraw-Hill Book Co, 1976, p 812.
3. Warkany J: "Congenital Malformations." Chicago:Year Book Medical Publishers, 1971, p 1309.
4. Bernstein L: Congenital atresia of the oval window. Arch Otolaryngol 83:43–47, 1966.
5. Hough JV: Malformations and anatomical variations seen in the middle ear during the operation for mobilization of the stapes. Laryngoscope 66:1337–1339, 1958.
6. Hough JV: Congenital malformations of the middle ear. Arch Otolaryngol 78:335–343, 1963.
7. Anson BJ: Development of the auditory ossicles. Laryngoscope 248:561–569, 1947.
8. Anson BJ, Hanson JS, Richany SF: Early embryology of the auditory

ossicles and associated structures in relation to certain anomalies observed clinically. Ann Otol Rhinol Laryngol 69:427–447, 1960.

9. Hanson R, Anson BJ, Strickland EM: Branchial sources of the auditory ossicles in man. II. Observations of embryonic states from 7 mm to 28 mm (CR length). Arch Otolaryngol 76:200–215, 1962.

10. Reagen FP: The role of the auditory sensory epithelium in the formation of the stapedial plate. J Exp Zool 23:85–108, 1917.

11. Simons EV: The effects of experimental unilateral anotia on skull development in the chick embryo. I. Introduction, technique, and preliminary results. Acta Morphol Neerl Scand 12:331–334, 1974.

12. Marovitz WF, Shapiro LJ: The distribution of phosphorylase activity in the otic capsule and ossicular chain of fetal and neonatal rats. Ann Otol Rhinol Laryngol 78:587–598, 1969.

13. Marovitz, WF, Proubsky ES: The distribution of phosphatases, mucopolysaccharides, and calcium in the otic capsule and ossicular chain of fetal and neonatal rats. Laryngoscope 81:273–296, 1971.

14. Jaskoll TF, Maderson PFA: A histological study of the development of the avian middle ear and tympanum. Anat Rec 190:177–200, 1978.

15. Jaskoll TF: "The Microscopic Anatomy and Dynamics of Avian and Mammalian Middle Ear Development." PhD thesis, City University of New York, 1978.

16. Jenkinson JW: The development of the ear bones in the mouse. J Anat Physiol 45:305–318, 1911.

17. Smith G: The middle ear and columella of birds. Q J Microsc Sci 48:11–22, 1904.

18. Stephens CB: Development of middle and inner ear in the golden hamster (*Mesocricetus auratus*). A detailed description to establish a norm for physiopathological study of congenital deafness. Acta Otolaryngol [Suppl] (Stockh) 296:1–51, 1972.

19. Romanoff AL: "The Avian Embryo." New York:Macmillan Co, 1960, p 1305.

20. Hamburger V, Hamilton HL: A series of normal stages in the development of the chick embryo. J Morphol 88:49–92, 1951.

21. Kalter H, Warkany J: Experimental production of congenital malformations in strains of inbred mice by hypervitaminosis A. Am J Pathol 38:1–21, 1961.

22. Wilson JG: "Environment and Birth Defects." New York:Academic Press, 1973, p 305.

23. Poswillo D: The pathogenesis of the Treacher Collins syndrome (mandibulofacial dysostosis). Br J Oral Surg 13:1–26, 1975.

24. Poswillo D: The pathogenesis of the first and second branchial arch syndrome. Oral Surg 35:302–328, 1973.

25. Poswillo D: Hemorrhage in development of the face. In Bergsma D (ed): "Morphogenesis and Malformation of Face and Brain." New York:Alan R Liss for The National Foundation-March of Dimes, BD:OAS XI(7):61–81, 1975.

26. Shenefelt RE: Morphogenesis of malformations in hamsters caused by retinoic acid: Relation to dose and stage of treatment. Teratology 5:103–118, 1972.

27. Ferguson MW: The teratogenic effects of 5-fluoro-2-desoxyuridine (FUDR) on the Wistar rat fetus, with particular reference to cleft palate. J Anat 126:37–47, 1978.

28. Singh G, Singh S, Padmanabhan R: Malformations of the ear induced by hypervitaminosis A in rat fetuses. Indian J Med Res 66:661–666, 1977.
29. Stivers FE, Steffek AJ, Yarrington CT: Effect of lathyrogens on developing midfacial structures of the rat. J Surg Res 11:415–420, 1971.
30. Altmann F: The ear in severe malformations of the head. Arch Otolaryngol 66:7–26, 1957.
31. Jaskoll TF, Melnick M, Slavkin HC: Unpublished data.
32. Jaskoll TF, Shah RM: Unpublished data.
33. Jaskoll TF, Maderson PFA, Weiner BE: The differentiation of the columella in avian embryos treated with hadacidin with some observations on other skeletal abnormalities. Teratology 18:321–332, 1978.
34. Romanoff AL, Romanoff AJ: "Pathogenesis of the Avian Embryo." New York:Wiley-Interscience, 1972, p 476.
35. Le Lievre CS: Rôle des cellules mésectodermiques issues des crêtes neurales céphaliques dans la formation des arcs branchiaux et du squelette viscéral. J Embryol Exp Morphol 31:453–477, 1974.
36. Le Lievre CS, Le Douarin NM: Mesenchymal derivatives of the neural crest: Analysis of chimaeric quail and chick embryos. J Embryol Exp Morphol 34:125–154, 1975.
37. Morriss GM: Abnormal cell migration as a possible factor in the genesis of vitamin A induced cranio-facial abnormalities. In Neubert E, Merker AS (eds): "New Approaches to the Evaluation of Abnormal Embryonic Development." Stuttgart:George Thieme, 1975, p 678–687.
38. Hassell JR, Greenberg JH, Johnston MC: Inhibition of cranial neural crest development by vitamin A in the cultured chick embryo. J Embryol Exp Morphol 39:267–271, 1977.
39. Hall BK: "Developmental and Cellular Skeletal Biology." New York:Academic Press, 1978, p 304.
40. Benoit JAA, Schowing J: Morphogenesis of the neurocranium. In Wolff E (ed): "Tissue Interactions during Organogenesis." New York:Gorden and Breach Publishers, 1970, p 105–129.
41. Coulombre AJ, Crelin ES: The role of the developing eye in the morphogenesis of the avian skull. Am J Phys Anthropol 16:25–37, 1958.
42. Leibel WS: The influence of the otic capsule in Ambrystomid skull formation. J Exp Zool 196:85–104, 1976.
43. Corsin J: Role des ebauches sensorielles au cours de la morphogenese du chondrocrane chez Pleurodeles waltlii Michah. Arch Anat Microsc Morphol Exp 61:47–59, 1972.
44. Jaskoll TF, Slavkin HC: Unpublished data.
45. Friedmann I, Hodges MG, Riddle PN: Organ culture of the mammalian and avian embryo otocyst. Ann Oto Rhinol Laryngol 86:371–380, 1977.
46. Van De Water TR, Maderson FPA, Jaskoll TF: The morphogenesis of the middle and external ear. In Gorlin R (ed): "Morphogenesis and Malformation of the Ear." New York:Alan R Liss for the March of Dimes Birth Defects Foundation, BD:OAS XVI(4):147–180, 1980.

Pathogenesis of Hereditary Inner Ear Abnormalities in Animals*

Robert J. Ruben, MD

Inherited deafness occurs in many different animals and is genetically heterogeneous. These animal models can serve to further our understanding of the disorder in man. This paper will summarize the results of studies in some of the animal models for hereditary deafness.

Deafness in the Hedlund white mink was first noted by Shakleford and Moore [1]. These animals respond to sound until the third or fourth week of life [2]. Early anatomic studies [3] showed degeneration of the organ of Corti, tectorial membrane, and Reissner membrane. Further examination of these animals [4–6] indicated that pathologic changes first occurred in the stria vascularis; changes then extended to the organ of Corti and finally to the saccule. These investigators suggested that the degeneration was due to a decrease in the vascularity of the stria vascularis which led to cell death of the organ of Corti and to collapse of the saccule.

The waltzing guinea pig was first found to be deaf by Ibsen and Risty [7]. Inheritance is as an autosomal dominant disorder, lethal in the homozygous state. The anatomic pathology was described by Lurie [8]. More recent studies [9–12] have shown that the organ of Corti in these

*Supported by grants from NIH (5 RO1 NSO8365–12), Deafness Research Foundation, March of Dimes Birth Defects Foundation (#1372), C.H.E.A.R., and the Manheimer Fund.

Birth Defects: Original Article Series, Volume XVI, Number 7, pages 29–34

animals develops and then degenerates. Electron micro-scopic examination reveals that degeneration begins at the cuticular plate at the top of the hair cells; degenera-tion is also found in the vestibular hair cells. The Type I vestibular hair cell was found to contain needle-shaped inclusion bodies which grow uncontrollably into dense bodies [13]. These inclusion bodies have been identified as actin.

Deafness in the white cat was first reported by Darwin [14] and is an autosomal dominant disorder. The condi-tion is associated with a white or partially white coat, blue and/or heterochromia irides. One or both ears may be affected. The lesion is progressive and its end state is degeneration of the cochlea and the saccule. The se-quence of cellular events, however, is not completely known [15, 16]. Transneuronal degeneration in these ani-mals has also been noted [17]. Pujol et al [18] have found a primary anterograde degeneration in the nerve fibers and ganglion of the acoustic nerve. These investigators noted that the same changes were not found in all ani-mals and suggested genetic heterogeneity.

Deafness in the Dalmation dog was first described by Rawitz [19]. The disorder is inherited as an autosomal dominant with considerable variation in expression: some animals have only one affected ear, while others have only a portion of an ear affected. Recent studies [20, 21] have demonstrated deafness in this animal to be due to cochlea-saccule degeneration. The lesion begins in the stria vascularis [22], with decrease in vascularity. The disease then sequentially effects the organ of Corti, Re-issner membrane, and finally the saccule.

Inherited deafness in the mouse has been studied since the beginning of the 20th century [23]. Yerkes [23] sum-marized the available data on these mice which were originally bred as children's pets in Japan. Today more than 30 different strains of deaf mice are known [24]. The shaker-1 mouse has been extensively studied and inherits deafness as an autosomal recessive disorder. The pathol-ogy and physiology of this animal have been described

[25–29]. There is degeneration of the organ of Corti and the saccule and atrophy in the stria vascularis. No changes, however, have been noted in the endocochlear potential. Electron microscopic examination of early degenerative changes in these animals noted changes within the hair cells.

The examples of inner ear degeneration of the cat, mink, guinea pig, dog, and mouse all have a common type of cellular mechanism. Development of the neural epithelium of the inner ear is normal in all of these animals and all have normal bony labyrinths. Several abnormal mechanisms which result in the degeneration of the organ of Corti have been suggested. These include abnormalities of the stria vascularis, and deposition of actin within the hair cells. Many different causes can result in premature death of the neural epithelial cells of the inner ear. The inner ear cannot grow new receptor cells as it is an end-state organ; neural epithelial cells cannot undergo further mitoses after the early embryologic development. In the mouse, the terminal mitosis for the neural epithelium of the cochlea is completed at approximately the 14th day of gestational life [30]. Thus, premature cell death would result in deafness. The biochemical abnormalities underlying early cell death are unknown. Heterogeneity should be expected. This type of pathology, early cell death with a normal bony labyrinth, is the most common pathology found both in animals and in man.

Another type of inner ear defect is found in the kreisler mouse. This is an autosomal recessive defect first noted as a result of an x-ray induced mutation by Hertwig [31]. The embryologic pathology of this animal has been associated with abnormalities of the neural tube [32] and cell cycle time [33]. The bony and membranous portions of the inner ear of the kreisler mouse are malformed. The extent of the malformation varies from animal to animal and from side to side. Deol has pointed out that the kreisler malformations may be secondary to abnormalities of the developing CNS [34, 35]. This hypothesis is supported by the embryologic evidence that the developing CNS is necessary for an orderly development of the inner ear [36]. Both the genetic studies of Deol and the embryologic studies indicate that the developing CNS does play a significant role in the orderly development of the normal inner ear, especially in regard to its anatomic form.

SUMMARY

There are many different genetic syndromes in animals which result in deafness. Two major types of inherited deafness are known. The most common in animals, including man, is that in which there is early cell death of the neural epithelium. This is found in the cat, dog, mink, guinea pig, and mouse.

The second type of inner ear deafness is associated with malformations of both the bony form of the inner ear and the neural epithelium. This type of deafness is that which is found in the kreisler mouse. It is also found in man, but appears to be less common than the early cell death in which there is no malformation of the bony labyrinth. This form of inherited deafness has been associated and may be secondary to genetic abnormalities of the developing CNS.

REFERENCES

1. Shakleford RM, Moore WB: Genetic basis of some white phenotypes in the ranch mink. J Hered 45:173–176, 1954.
2. Flottorp G, Foss I: Development of hearing in the hereditarily deaf white mink (Hedlund) and normal mink (standard) and subsequent deterioration of the auditory response of a Hedlund mink. Acta Otolaryngol (Stockh) 87:16–27, 1979.
3. Saunders LZ: Histopathology of hereditary congenital deafness in the white mink. Path Vet 2:256–263, 1965.
4. Hilding DA, Sugiura A, Niki Y: The deaf white mink: Electromicroscopic study of the inner ear. Ann Otol Rhinol Laryngol 67:647–663, 1967.
5. Sugiura A, Hilding DA: The deaf white mink: Electron microscopic study of the inner ear. Acta Otolaryngol (Stockh) 69:126–137, 1970.
6. Sugiura A, Hilding DA: Stria vascularis of the deaf Hedlund mink. Light and electron microscopic studies of vascular insufficiency. Acta Otolaryngol (Stockh) 69:160–171, 1970.
7. Ibsen LH, Risty TK: A new character in guinea pigs, waltzing. Anat Rec 44:294, 1929.

8. Lurie MH: Studies of the waltzing guinea pig. Laryngoscope 49:559, 1939.

9. Ernstson S: Cochlear morphology in a strain of the waltzing guinea pig. Acta Otolaryngol (Stockh) 71:469–482, 1971.

10. Ernstson S: Cochlear physiology in a hair cell population in a strain of waltzing guinea pig. Acta Otolaryngol [Suppl] (Stockh) 297:1–24, 1972.

11. Ernstson S: Heredity in a strain of the waltzing guinea pig. Acta Otolaryngol (Stockh) 69:358–362, 1970.

12. Ernstson S, Lundquist PG, Wedenberg E, Wersall J: Morphological changes in the vestibular hair cell strain of the waltzing guinea pig. Acta Otolaryngol (Stockh) 67:521–534, 1969.

13. Flock A, Cheung H, Wersall J: Pathological action of vestibular hair cells of the waltzing guinea pig. Adv Otorhinolaryngol 25:12–16, 1979.

14. Darwin C: "Origin of the Species." London:Murray, 1859.

15. Bosher SK, Hallpike FRS: Observations on the histological features, development and pathogenesis of the inner ear degeneration of the deaf white cat. Proc R Soc Lond [Biol] 162:147–170, 1965.

16. Mair IW: Hereditary deafness in the white cat. Acta Otolaryngol [Suppl] (Stockh) 314:1–48, 1973.

17. West CD, Harrison JM: Transneuronal cell atrophy in the congenitally deaf white cat. J Comp Neurol 151:377–398, 1973.

18. Pujol R, Rebillard M, Rebillard G: Primary neural disorders in the deaf white cat cochlea. Acta Otolaryngol (Stockh) 83:59–64, 1977.

19. Rawitz B: Morphol Arbiet 6:545–554, 1896.

20. Anderson H, Henricson B, Lundquist PG, Wedenberg E, Wersall J: Genetic hearing impairment in the Dalmation dog. An audiometric, genetic and morphologic study in 53 dogs. Acta Otolaryngol [Suppl] (Stockh) 232:1–34, 1968.

21. Hudson WR, Ruben RJ: Hereditary deafness in the Dalmation dog. Arch Otolaryngol 75:213–219, 1962.

22. Johnson LG, Hawkins JE Jr, Muraski AA, Preston RE: Vascular anatomy and pathology of the cochlea in Dalmation dogs. In Darin de Lorenzo AJ (ed): "Vascular Disorders and Hearing Defect." Baltimore:University Park Press, 1973, pp 249–296.

23. Yerkes RM: "The Dancing Mouse as Studies in Animal Behavior." New York:Macmillan, 1907.

24. Alben PL, Katz DD (eds): Inbred and genetically defined strains of laboratory animals. I. Mouse and rat. "Biological Handbooks," Vol III. Bethesda:Federation of American Societies for Experimental Biology, 1979.

25. Brown PG, Ruben RJ: Endocochlear potential in the shaker-1 mouse. Acta Otolaryngol (Stockh) 68:14–20, 1969.

26. Kikuchi K, Hilding DA: The defective organ of Corti in the shaker-1 mice. Acta Otolaryngol (Stockh) 60:287–303, 1965.

27. Mikaelian D, Alford BR, Ruben RJ: Cochlear potentials and VIII nerve action potentials in normal and genetically deaf mice. Ann Otol 74:146–158, 1965.

28. Mikaelian DO, Ruben RJ: Hearing degeneration in shaker-1 mouse. Arch Otolaryngol 80:418–430, 1964.

29. Sato Y, Sato M, Ruben RJ: Oxygen consumption of the membranous cochlea and other tissues in shaker-1 (sh-1/sh-1) and normal (CBA-J/CBA-J) mice. Acta Otolaryngol (Stockh) 68:239–242, 1969.

30. Ruben RJ: Development of the inner ear of the mouse: A radioautographic study of terminal mitoses. Acta Otolaryngol [Suppl] (Stockh) 220:1–44, 1967.
31. Hertwig P: Neue Mutation und Koppelungsgruppen bie der Hausmaous. Z Indukt Abstamm Vererb L 80:220–246, 1942.
32. Deol MS: The abnormalities of the inner ear in the kreisler mouse. J Embryol Exp Morphol 12:475–490, 1964.
33. Ruben RJ: Development and cell kinetics of the kreisler (kr/kr) mouse. Laryngoscope 83:1440–1468, 1973.
34. Deol MS: Influence of the neural tube on differentiation of the inner ear of the mammalian embryo. Nature 209:2, 1966.
35. Deol MS: Inherited diseases of the inner ear in man in light of studies on the mouse. J Med Genet 5:137–158, 1968.
36. Van De Water TR, Li CW, Ruben RJ, Shea CA: Ontogenic aspects of mammalian inner ear development. In Gorlin R (ed): "Morphogenesis and Malformation of the Ear." New York:Alan R Liss for the March of Dimes Birth Defects Foundation, BD:OAS XVI(4):5–46, 1980.

Nonsyndromic Deafness*

Walter E. Nance, MD, PhD

The precise interaction of hundreds—perhaps thousands—of gene pairs must be required to form a normal human ear. Defects in any one of this large number of genes or gene pairs can lead to hearing loss. The recognition of the extensive etiologic heterogeneity that exists among the genetic and environmental causes of deafness has been the outstanding achievement of clinical research on human deafness syndromes during the past quarter century.

The classification of hereditary deafness syndromes based on the pleiotropic effects of the relevant mutations has been the most successful approach to the recognition of heterogeneity and has resulted in the delineation of more than 150 clinical entities which are at times associated with hearing loss [1–4]. However, clinical nosology has its limits, and in human genetics it is frequently not possible to distinguish between allelic and nonallelic variation by clinical criteria alone. Subtle phenotypic distinctions require sound clinical judgment; they may be idiosyncratic to single pedigrees and can be influenced by unrecognized ascertainment biases.

Audiologic findings, either in affected patients or heterozygous carriers, have also been used with some success to distinguish different forms of hereditary deafness [4, 5]. Most, but not all, patients with profound genetic sensorineural hearing loss may have been deaf at or before birth. Among cases with residual hearing at birth there

*Supported in part by grants from the March of Dimes Birth Defects Foundation, the Retinitis Pigmentosa Foundation, and USPHS AM/MD-25786. Paper No. 96 from the Department of Human Genetics of the Medical College of Virginia.

Birth Defects: Original Article Series, Volume XVI, Number 7, pages 35–46
© 1980 March of Dimes Birth Defects Foundation

may be considerable variation in the age of onset, rate of progression, and ultimate severity of the audiologic deficit [6]. The retention of almost any degree of hearing during the prelingual period can profoundly improve the ability of an infant to communicate with the environment. It could account for the great variation in linguistic skills of deaf children who, when tested at a later date, appear to have hearing losses of comparable severity. Whether heterozygous carriers of recessive genes for deafness ever show minor audiologic abnormalities has never been rigorously tested [7]. It is highly plausible to expect that manifesting heterozygotes must exist at some of the many loci that contribute to recessive deafness. As a practical matter, audiologic studies are routinely recommended for the parents of children with profound hearing loss and these test results are considered with the pedigree data and clinical findings in the overall evaluation and counseling. Although audiologic findings have probably not been adequately exploited, their contribution to the nosology of deafness is subject to the same limitations as other clinical criteria.

Genetic linkage studies are also a very powerful approach to the recognition of genetic heterogeneity; however, such studies have been almost completely ignored in the delineation of the hereditary deafness syndromes. With the exception of the X-linked forms of deafness and the putative linkage of Waardenburg syndrome to the ABO locus on chromosome 9 [8], no other deafness syndrome has yet been mapped.

The high degree of assortative mating that exists among deaf people provides abundant opportunities for the definition of heterogeneity in recessive deafness syndromes through yet another approach: the analysis of in vivo complementation. Figure 1 shows schematically how the observation of critical matings among affected individuals in several kindreds could ultimately lead to the identification of complementation groups. Detailed comparisons of groups of affected individuals defined in this manner might then permit the recognition of other characteristic clinical, genetic, audiologic, or biochemical dif-

HYPOTHETICAL PEDIGREE
DEMONSTRATING COMPLEMENTATION

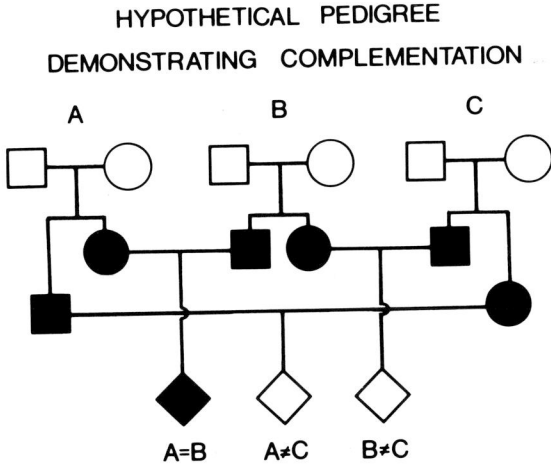

Fig. 1. Hypothetical pedigree demonstrating complementation.

ferences. Most contemporary studies of hereditary deafness have employed truncate selection through affected offspring; no systematic attempt has been made to use complex interrelationships of this type in any large body of pedigree data. Although valid inferences could be drawn from an analysis of pedigree data alone, the power of any such study would obviously be greatly enhanced by the availability of accurate clinical observations. This principle is well illustrated by a deaf-by-deaf mating shown in Figure 2 in which both sons were also deaf. Since all grandparents had normal hearing, one would have been tempted to assume that both parents had the same form of recessive deafness, leading to noncomplementation in the offspring. The father had Usher syndrome (Type II) with severe visual impairment; because of his understanding of the recessive inheritance of Usher syndrome, the possibility that his sons and wife might also have Usher syndrome and therefore be at risk for the later development of retinitis pigmentosa and visual impairment was a matter of great concern to him. Fortunately, the mother and sons were examined and found to have onychodystrophy. This family is the second example

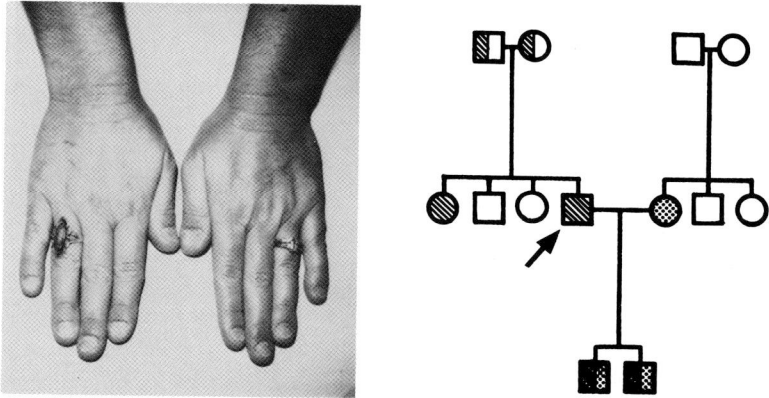

Fig. 2. Pedigree showing mating between a hearing-impaired male with Usher syndrome and a woman with onychodystrophy. Note the thin friable spoon-shaped nails on the left. Both sons had similar nails and hearing impairment.

of dominant transmission of onychodystrophy and deafness among the 8 families reported [9] and provides a satisfying and reassuring explanation for the pedigree.

Finally, segregation analysis [10] provides a useful method of summarizing a large body of pedigree data in terms of a few informative population parameters. This technique attempts to resolve families into high risk and low risk, or sporadic groups. The sporadic cases are those in which there is a negligible recurrence risk and in the case of deafness might include hearing loss due to environmental factors, such as rubella or ototoxic drugs, as well as new mutations in which familial recurrence within the proband sibship would be very unlikely. The proportion of sporadic cases is measured by the variable x. The familial cases which constitute a proportion $(1 - x)$ of all affected subjects are those in which there is a substantial recurrence risk. This method of analysis actually makes no assumption about the cause of any observed evidence for familial aggregation; it is only when the magnitude of the recurrent risk, or segregation ratio, p, in various mating types corresponds to our preconceptions for a mendelian trait that we are tempted to infer a genetic etiology. The final parameter, π, is the ascertainment probability, that is to say, the probability that an affected individual is a proband or index case. The value of π can range from nearly zero (single selection) to one (complete selection). The former would imply that every family would have only a single proband while the latter occurs when every family is independently discovered through each affected individual. Although the value of π is of no intrinsic genetic interest, it must be included in the analysis to avoid estimation bias. Segregation analysis can also be used to search for secular trends in the etiology of deafness as well as to provide empiric risk data in cases where the diagnosis of a specific deafness syndrome cannot be made. The following results of a comparative study of 3 large data sets illustrate this method of analysis.

The first sample of families was based on data collected as part of a National Survey by the Office of Demographic Studies at Gallaudet College in 1969 and reported by Rose et al [10, 11]. Pedigree information was obtained on 12,661 nuclear families which included a deaf proband and at least one other sib for a grand total of 16,471 deaf and 33,294 hearing children. In Table 1, the results of separate segregation analyses of the hearing-by-hearing and deaf-by-hearing matings are summarized. The analyses were performed using a modification of Morton's Segran Program [12] with π fixed at 0.325, a value derived from a preliminary analysis of the distribution of probands among affected subjects. The hearing-by-hearing matings were divided into 2 groups: those in which there was a remote family history of deafness in a more distant relative, such as a grandparent or cousin, and a much larger group in which there was no such history. In both subsets, the null hypothesis that all cases were determined by fully penetrant recessive genes was rejected. This hypothesis was tested by setting $p = 0.25$, the value that would be expected assuming recessive inheritance, and $x = 0$, the value expected if all cases were genetic. The large values of χ^2 indicate that these assumptions do

TABLE 1. Results of Segregation Analysis in Hearing-by-Hearing and Deaf-by-Hearing Matings in National Survey*

Type of Mating & Hypothesis Tested	No. of Sibships	No. of Children		χ_p^2	χ_x^2
		Deaf	Hearing		
Hearing-by-Hearing					
Positive family history					
H_0:p=0.25, x=0.0	1,391	2,142	3,496	96.97	103.85
H_1:p=0.25, x=$\hat{x}$=0.203	1,391	2,142	3,496	0.05	—
Negative family history					
H_0:p=0.25, x=0.0	10,509	12,712	28,739	5,298.63	5,832.79
H_1:p=0.25, x=$\hat{x}$=0.605	10,509	12,712	28,739	1.93	—
Deaf-by-Hearing					
Positive family history					
H_0:p=0.50, x=0.0	106	324	325	53.44	116.19
H_1:p=$\hat{p}$=0.31, x=0.0	106	324	325	—	1.12
Negative family history					
H_0:p=0.50, x=0.0	94	154	219	100.72	236.05
H_1:p=$\hat{p}$=0.21, x=0.0	94	154	219	—	0.27

*Adapted from Rose et al [10].

not account adequately for the observed data. However, the alternative hypotheses that about 20% and 60% of the cases were sporadic in the positive and negative family history cases, respectively, while the remainder were fully penetrant recessives, provide an excellent explanation for the data. In this trial, the best fitting or maximum likelihood values of x were used for the test. These findings immediately suggest that the elicitation of a remote family history of deafness has a profound influence on the prior probability that a proband has a recessive rather than a sporadic form of deafness. In the deaf-by-hearing matings, it seemed reasonable to assume that all families with an affected child represented genetic cases (ie $x = 0$). However, we observed again that a history of other deaf antecedents had an effect, this time on the estimated penetrance of the dominant gene in question which was found to be 62% in the presence of and 42% in the absence of a remote family history of deafness. Similar analyses were performed on 2 other data sets. The first analysis was of a sample of 2,335 informative families, including a total of 18,609 individuals most of whom were

TABLE 2. Classification of Deafness: Comparison of Survey Estimates*

| Survey | Year | No. of Matings | Deaf Offspring | | | Genetic Types | |
			Total	Percent Sporadic	Percent Genetic	Percent Dominant	Percent Recessive
Fay Survey	1900	2,335	3,483	45.1	54.9	12.0	88.0
National Survey	1969	12,665	16,482	49.3	50.7	14.4	85.6
Gallaudet Survey	1973	486	749	23.8	76.2	22.2	77.8

*Adapted from Rose et al [10].

ascertained through matings among the deaf by Fay at the turn of the century [13]. The second sample reported by Nance et al [14] included data on 1,755 offspring in 486 informative pedigrees collected from the parents of students at Gallaudet College in 1973.

Table 2 summarizes the results of the 3 studies. Almost half the cases in the National Survey were estimated to be genetic and half sporadic. In the Fay study, a greater proportion were estimated to be genetic. In view of the dramatic advances that have been made in the prevention of many environmental causes of deafness it might have been anticipated that the proportion of genetic cases would have increased during the past 70 years. Evidently, there must have been a concomitant decrease in the number of genetic cases. It seems possible this decrease may have occurred as a consequence of the breaking up of inbred isolates; the modest decline in the estimated proportion of recessive cases is consistent with this view.

Alternatively, it may well be that the Gallaudet Survey is a more appropriate group for comparative purposes, since Fay's study was based primarily on married deaf adults while the National Survey included many severely affected children, those with rubella for example, who may never contribute substantially to the marital pool of deaf adults. In any event, in the Gallaudet Survey, a startling high proportion of cases—85%—were estimated to be genetic. The increased proportion of genetic cases in the high achieving Gallaudet student population may also indicate that genetic causes of deafness are less frequently associated with other neurologic impairment.

The members of the large cohort of children with rubella deafness who were born during the 1964 epidemic provide an explicit example of this phenomenon since these are included in the National Survey, but not the Gallaudet Study. Whether the increased proportion of dominant deafness among students at Gallaudet reflects higher average levels of educational attainment among deaf students who have at least one deaf parent, or reflects an aggregate biologic difference between dominant and recessive forms of deafness, remains conjectural.

The parameter estimates for π, p, and x that are derived for the relevant mating types in the first 2 sets of data may be used, as shown in Table 3, to obtain empiric risk estimates that are appropriate for genetic counseling [15]. In a normal-by-normal mating with a single affected child, the probability that the next child will be affected varies, depending upon whether there is a remote history of deafness. As more normal sibs are born into the family, the probability that the case was genetic in the first place decreases and the estimated recurrence risk therefore declines. If there are 2 affected children, if a history of consanguinity can be elicited, or if a specific recessive syndrome can be diagnosed, the appropriate risk figure would, of course, be 25%.

Deaf-by-normal matings may come for counseling either before or after the birth of an affected child. The empiric risk for their having a first affected child is only 6.7% and declines to 1.0% after the birth of 4 normal children. Dominant inheritance can be assumed to be the hereditary mechanism in families who have already had at least one affected child. However, the risk of their having another deaf child is less than 50% because of reduced penetrance. This result is consistent with the findings for many recognized dominant forms of deafness, such as Waardenburg syndrome, which show marked variation in expressivity and incomplete penetrance for deafness [4].

Deaf-by-deaf matings are more complex. Even if both parents have recessive deafness, they may be capable of

TABLE 3. Recurrence Risk of Subsequent Deaf Offspring in Various Matings*

Mating Types	Number of Deaf Offspring	Number of Tested Offspring (N)					
		0	1	2	3	4	5
Normal-by-normal							
Positive family history	1	—	0.200	0.187	0.172	0.156	0.138
Negative family history	1	—	0.098	0.082	0.067	0.054	0.043
Deaf-by-normal							
All normal children	0	0.067	0.043	0.026	0.016	0.010	0.006
At least 1 deaf child	>0	—	0.408	0.408	0.408	0.408	0.408
Deaf-by-deaf							
All normal children	0	0.097	0.041	0.029	0.020	0.014	0.010
All deaf children	N	0.097	0.617	0.799	0.918	0.966	0.990
Deaf and normal children	>0>N	—	—	0.325	0.325	0.325	0.325

*Adapted from Bieber and Nance [15].

producing only normal children if the mutations they carry are complementary (ie nonallelic). On the other hand, if the parents have the same type of recessive deafness, then all their children will be expected to be affected. Finally, several situations, including the presence of a dominant gene for deafness in one of the parents, could lead to the birth of both deaf and normal children. Prior to the birth of any children, the empiric risk for deaf-by-deaf matings is only about 9.7%, which testifies to the large number of recessive loci that contribute to profound deafness. The phenotype of the first child has a dramatic effect on the risk estimate for subsequent children. If the child is deaf, there is a sixfold increase in the empiric risk for the next child, and the risk rapidly approaches 100% as additional deaf children are born into the family. If the child is normal, however, the risk falls to 4.1% and continues to decline as additional normal children are born. Finally, if the couple has had both deaf and normal children, it is clearly a segregating mating and the empiric recurrent risk for this situation in our data set turned out to be 32.5%.

These estimates are based on what is probably the largest sample of pedigrees of a single clinical phenotype that has ever been subjected to segregation analysis and are appropriate for cases in which a definite etiology cannot be established; however, caution should be advised in their use. The analyses were based on all cases

in which adequate family history data were available, and
no attempt was made to remove cases attributable either
to obvious genetic syndromes or known environmental
cases. The rubella syndrome is at least one cause of
congenital deafness whose incidence can vary tremen-
dously from year to year, thus confounding any meaning-
ful estimate of the overall proportions of genetic and
environmental deafness. Our data set from the National
Survey included children born in the 1964 pandemic. The
potential effect of this epidemic on our estimates is
shown in Figure 3 which gives the distribution of birth
dates for the 147 current students at the Maryland School
for the Deaf who have a diagnosis of congenital rubella
syndrome. There was a dramatic increase in the incidence of rubella deafness in the winter of 1964, with
more than 10 times as many cases born during that winter as were born during the seasonal peaks of the preced-
ing and following winters. There is a hint in the data from
the Maryland School for the Deaf that the performance
scores of the rubella children born after November 1964
are lower than those born before November; this difference could be explained by an earlier exposure during
pregnancy to the teratogenic virus. In any event, epidemic causes of deafness can greatly alter the risk figures
used above; these figures should, ideally, be based on
sequential analyses by year of birth. The annual collection and segregation analysis of pedigree data from deaf
probands would provide a highly sensitive method of
monitoring secular changes in the etiology of deafness
and could lead to the early detection of unexpected epi-
demics of deafness caused, for example, by other viruses
or possibly by the introduction of new ototoxic drugs or
pollutants into the environment.

In practice, the risk table is used as a starting point for
counseling in cases of deafness in which a specific genetic
or environmental cause cannot be determined. The parents are told that the data are based solely on an analysis
of the family histories of a large number of individuals
like themselves, and that if nothing about them other than

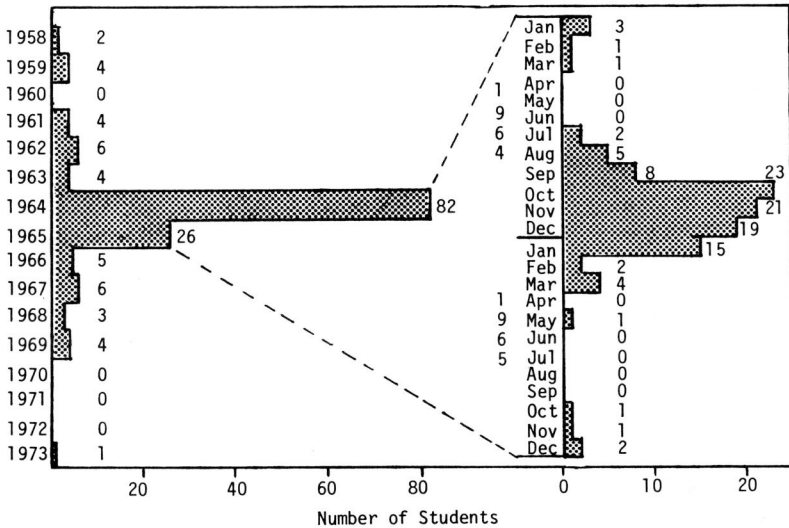

Fig. 3. Distribution of birth dates for 147 rubella students at the Maryland School for the Deaf by year and by month for the 1964-1965 cohort.

their family history is known, the tables would provide an appropriate risk figure. However, if there is no hint of an environmental cause such as rubella or perinatal complication, or if the parents of a hearing-impaired child have minor audiologic abnormalties, the figures in the table would be quoted as a minimum risk with the maximum being 25%. On the other hand, if there is a suspicious but equivocal history of an environmental etiology, the appropriate entry could be used as a maximum risk figure. In this way it is possible to incorporate the subtle clinical impressions formed during the evaluation into the counseling but still retain a factual basis for the risk figure used. When accompanied by discussion of the ubiquity of recessive genes, most hearing parents of deaf children seem to respond well to this approach to genetic counseling.

ACKNOWLEDGMENTS

A large number of present and former students, colleagues, and associates assisted in the collection and analysis of the data described in this paper. I would like to acknowledge especially the contributions of Drs. Susan Rose, P. M. Conneally, Joann Boughman, Judy Z. Miller, A. C. McLeod, and R. Trybus, as well as Frederick Bieber, G. Fellendorf, Patricia Fox and Anne Sweeney.

REFERENCES

1. McKusick, VA: "Mendelian Inheritance in Man," 5th Ed. Baltimore:The Johns Hopkins University Press, 1978.
2. Fraser GR: "The Causes of Profound Deafness in Childhood." Baltimore:The Johns Hopkins University Press, 1976.
3. Konigsmark BW, Gorlin RJ: "Genetic and Metabolic Deafness." Philadelphia:WB Saunders, 1976.
4. Nance WE, McConnell FE: Status and prospects of research in hereditary deafness. Adv Hum Genet 4:173–250, 1973.
5. McLeod AC, Sweeney A, McConnell FE, Kemker J, Nance WE, Webb WE: Autosomal recessive sensorineural deafness: A comparison of two kindreds. South Med J 66:141, 1973.
6. Nance WE, Sweeney A: Genetic factors in deafness of early life. Otolaryngol Clin North Am 8:19–48, 1975.
7. McLeod AC, McConnell FE, Sweeney A, Cooper MC, Nance WE: Clinical variation in Usher's syndrome. Arch Otolaryngol 94:321–334, 1971.
8. Arias S, Mota M, deYanez A, Bolivar M: Probable loose linkage between the ABO locus and Waardenburg syndrome. Humangenetik 27:145–149, 1975.
9. Bieber FR, Nance WE: Onycho-osteodystrophy and sensorineural deafness: Report of a new case (Abstract) XIV Int. Cong. of Genet. Moscow:Publishing Office "Nauka," 1978, pp 311.
10. Rose SP, Conneally PM, Nance WE: Genetic analysis of childhood deafness. In Bess FH (ed): "Childhood Deafness." New York:Grune & Stratton, 1977, pp 19–35.
11. Rose SP: "Genetic Studies of Profound Prelingual Deafness." PhD Thesis, Indiana University, 1975.
12. Morton NE: Genetic tests under incomplete ascertainment. Am J Hum Genet 11:1–16, 1959.
13. Fay EA: "Marriages of the Deaf in America." Washington:Gibson Bros., 1898.
14. Nance WE, Rose SP, Conneally PM, Miller JZ: Opportunities for genetic counseling through institutional ascertainment of affected probands. In Lubs HA, de la Cruz F (eds): "Genetic Counseling." New York:Raven Press, 1977.
15. Bieber FR, Nance WE: Hereditary hearing loss. In Jackson L, Schimke N (eds): "Clinical Genetics:A Source Book for Physicians." New York:John Wiley & Sons, 1979, pp 443–461.

Central Deafness: Fact or Fiction?

Charles I. Berlin, PhD

INTRODUCTION

Central hearing loss was predicted and even diagnosed before reliable tools for its measurement were available. However, those who made this diagnosis, as well as those who denied the existence of central hearing loss, were handicapped by the limited tools available for its verification and measurement.

For many years, the most common tools available for the measurement of central hearing loss were: 1) pure-tone audiometry, in which patients were requested to respond voluntarily to pure tones; 2) Speech Reception Threshold (SRT), in which patients were asked to respond to two-syllable words; 3) monosyllabic word discrimination tests, in which patients were asked to identify single-syllable words at high intensities; and 4) Galvanic Skin Response (GSR) audiometry, in which patients were presented a pure tone coupled with a shock in order to condition a change in skin resistance.

Because none of the few tools then available for measurement of central hearing loss was universally acceptable, intuition was often the major method for diagnosis of central hearing problems. Clinicians who diagnosed central hearing loss frequently found their rationale, proof, and management questioned. Unfortunately, during this period negative evidence for the existence of central hearing loss mounted faster than the positive evidence.

Although central hearing loss is a rare phenomenon, methods are now available for its measurement. There are some excellent behavioral methods [1]. However, with the judicious use of Auditory Brainstem Response (ABR), electrocochleography, and transcranial and ipsilat-

Birth Defects: Original Article Series, Volume XVI, Number 7, pages 47—57

erally elicited middle-ear muscle reflexes, certain forms of central dysfunction may be studied physiologically. This paper will review some of the negative and positive evidence for the existence of central hearing loss and present case material and experimental material which further confirm its existence.

NEGATIVE EVIDENCE FOR THE EXISTENCE OF CENTRAL HEARING LOSS

Clinicians who viewed the auditory system as a series of linear telephone cables often argued that central hearing loss did not exist because patients with known lesions of various portions of the rostral brainstem and cortex did not have audiometric losses. It is now known that even in hemispherectomies, or patients with bilateral temporal-lobe lesions, no substantial loss in the pure-tone audiogram can be recorded [2,3].

Central hearing loss was often assumed in adult patients with good pure-tone perception but unexpectedly poor speech perception in one or both ears. This diagnosis required that the patient be able to participate in speech perception tasks. Very few adult patients met this requirement; those who did almost always had caudal brainstem lesions. The diagnosis of central hearing loss in the nonverbal child was based on apparent ability to respond to faint environmental sounds with failure to comprehend speech [4]. Unfortunately, many children were misdiagnosed as having central hearing loss when their peripheral losses were of the shape and type that permitted the detection of clicks or noises but prohibited the comprehension of speech. The following acoustic rules conspired to make this misdiagnosis not only likely, but common: 1) In most peripheral sensorineural losses, the high frequencies are more poorly perceived than the low frequencies. However, there is evidence of a type of loss that operates in the opposite direction [5]. 2) When any signal is gated on abruptly, it tends to have a broad spectrum.

Thus, when clinicians used what they thougnt to be high frequency noisemakers to assess a child's responsiveness to high frequency sounds, the child responded to the low frequency portion of the broad acoustic spectrum generated by the brief onset rather than the intended high frequency stimuli. Thus, children with sloping hearing loss responded to noises but could not perceive speech and so were misdiagnosed as having central losses [3].

Galvanic Skin Response (GSR) audiometry, developed in the late 1940s and early 1950s at the Johns Hopkins Medical Institutions [6], potentially allowed the diagnostician to evaluate how much and what portion of various signals were reaching a patient's conscious awareness. In a select number of adult patients GSR audiometry probably worked this way [7]. However, problems with conditioning criteria, criteria for the acceptance of a true response, and the separation and analysis of false-positive vs false-negative responses created difficulties even with cooperative adults.

Many clinicians were often unable or unwilling to acquire GSR data needed from young children. Data collected were frequently inaccurate. Because children with both serious neurologic problems and sensory hearing loss could rarely be conditioned, they were misdiagnosed as having normal peripheral hearing. Tragically, such misdiagnosis often brought denial of a hearing aid.

POSITIVE EVIDENCE FOR THE EXISTENCE OF CENTRAL HEARING LOSS

Although central hearing loss is rare, evidence of its existence appears in the literature [8–11]. Two examples are particularly noteworthy. Landau et al [12], in what is now considered a landmark paper, presented a patient who had been considered to be deaf but ultimately responded normally to pure-tone audiometry and had adequate speech reception thresholds. Although the patient had normal intelligence he did not acquire speech and language adequately. At 10 days of age this white male was noted to have a cardiac murmur and to be cyanotic. He was toilet trained at 18 months, but did not sit until 14 months, and did not walk until 5 years. He was seen at the Johns Hopkins Hospital Cardiac Clinic at 6 years of age where transposition of the great vessels was noted and a diagnosis of a Taussig-Bing syndrome transposition complex was made.

The patient was seen the same year at the Central Institute for the Deaf. Normal speech detection and noise detection thresholds between 5 and 10 dB were obtained under earphones and in the sound field. However, he did not comprehend spoken language. Communication consisted of facial expressions and gestures accompanied by vocalizations that varied appropriately in pitch, inflection, and volume with the meaning he seemed to be trying to convey. He occasionally included appropriate single words. Although the psychologist reported the child's behavior indicated at least normal intelligence, an IQ of 78 was obtained on the Advanced Performance Scale.

After a year of training as an "aphasic child," repeated testing indicated an IQ of 97 using the Advanced Performance Scale. He had a functional reading, writing, and speaking vocabulary of at least 175 words. He had learned simple 4 to 6 sentence descriptive stories and could recite them from memory. He could also use learned sequences to answer rote questions. He could comprehend oral language when spoken slowly and with a definite pause after each word, but could only understand familiar expressions when spoken at a normal rate.

In December 1955, at 10 years of age, the patient became ill with mumps and died suddenly, presumably because of cardiac complications. The autopsy confirmed the cardiac syndrome diagnosis but the autopsy report on the central nervous system was of particular interest:

> The brain weighed 1150 grams and an external examination revealed no abnormality of the vessels at the base. The anterior portion of the brain was normal size and configuration but posteriorly, there was a bilateral loss of cortical substance starting from the inferior and posterior margins of the central sulci anteriorly, and extending backwards along the course of the insulae and Sylvian fissures towards the occipital lobe on each side. The gyri of the posterior portion of the parietal temporal and occipital lobes bilaterally were reduced in size, and increased numbers of convolutions were present. There were no abnormalities anterior to the central sulci, but posterior to this region, there was

atrophy of both white and gray matter of the insulae, their operculae, and the tissue immediately behind, extending into the occipital lobes.

In the brainstem, *the normally distinct medial geniculate structures closely related to the lateral geniculate nuclei and the cerebral peduncles were difficult to identify. Although it is not possible to say there was complete atrophy of the medial geniculate nuclei, it was obvious that they were severely degenerated. Both pyramidal tracts were degenerated along their ventral margins in the medulla. Both auditory nerves were histologically intact. The inner ear structures were not examined.* (italics added)

In summary, this patient had "bilateral old infarctions in the Sylvian regions, and severe retrograde degeneration in the medial geniculate nuclei. Language function, therefore, appears to have been subserved by pathways other than the primary auditory thalamocortical projection system."

Jerger et al [13] reported a 21-year-old patient who had suffered 2 cerebral hemisphere infarctions. This study is important for two reasons. First, the patient demonstrated the reality of "cortical deafness." Second, premorbid routine audiometry was available as an operating baseline. The patient, a member of the United States Air Force, had a normal pure-tone air conduction audiogram prior to his induction into military service. On admission for his second infarction, he had a flat 60–85 dB hearing loss at all frequencies in both ears. Three months later there had been some recovery, and although his hearing was essentially normal in the speech frequencies, a bilateral, high frequency loss which was more severe in the right ear remained. Speech understanding was impaired in both ears with the poorest performance in the right ear. Loudness discrimination was normal in the left ear but severely impaired in the right ear. Perception of auditory temporal order was severely impaired in both ears. Attempts at evoking auditory responses physiologically were fruitless from 100 msec onward with a bandpass of 0.2–12.0 Hz. Early evoked potentials, such as the ABR and the so-called middle evoked potentials were not studied.

Failure to obtain the late electroencephalogram (EEG) response in a patient who definitely hears pure-tone signals clearly indicates the existence of a central auditory deficit. Although this patient has not come to autopsy, the EEG results, brain-scan results, and arteriographic studies all successfully localized the lesions to the subcortical structures subtending both left and right temporal lobes. The authors conclude that the patient had occlusion of the terminal branches of the middle cerebral artery on each side at two different times resulting in a bilateral, partial, cerebral hemisphere infarction, maximally affecting the temporal lobes and producing the clinical picture of cortical deafness.

ABR is the most productive of the modern electrophysiologic tools. Wave-form recordings generated by this response (Fig. 1) represent synchronous discharges of first- through sixth-order onset-sensitive neurons in the central auditory system. While the source of the serial discharges is disputed, the nature, latencies, and synchrony of the normal ABR have been documented [14–20].

A technique for using the ABR to examine binaural (2-ear central) interaction involves recording the ABR to right-ear stimulation and to left-ear stimulation, and then adding them [21]. Then a binaural response is obtained and the sum of the 2 monaural responses is subtracted from the binaural response. The resulting difference potential is used as an index of binaural central interaction (Fig. 2). The rationale for such a procedure is derived from work by Webster and Webster [10, 22] and others [23, 24] who have shown that a peripheral, conductive hearing loss, and/or auditory deprivation leads to poor maintenance of certain nuclei in the caudal brainstem.

The following 2 cases illustrate central anomalies identified using modern electrophysiologic techniques. It is not yet known if the physiologic results obtained are pathognomonic for the diagnosis or simply fortuitous.

A 2-year old, referred because of failure to develop verbal language, was identified as deaf. Developmental milestones, aside from lack of speech and lack of re-

sponse to auditory stimuli, appeared normal. Tympanometry was normal and no transcranial reflexes to acoustic
stimuli were observed. On the basis of these findings the
child received a hearing aid but was balking at its use.

I   II III IV V

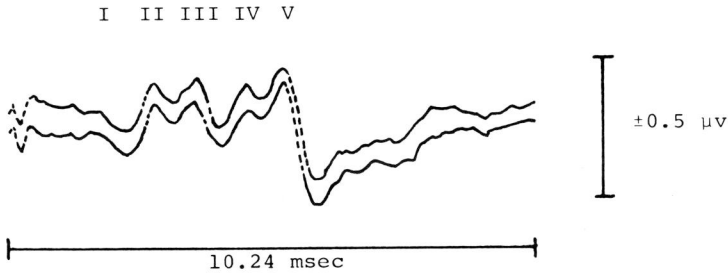

±0.5 µv

10.24 msec

Fig. 1.   An ABR (2 superimposed samples) from a normal human subject.

10.24 msec

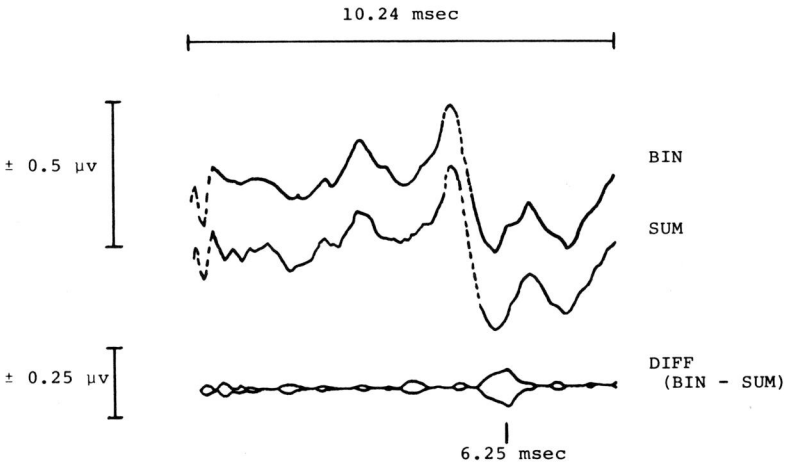

± 0.5 µv

BIN

SUM

± 0.25 µv

DIFF
(BIN - SUM)

6.25 msec

FIGURE 2

Fig. 2.   A binaural interaction component from a normal human subject. Trace
1 represents the ABR from binaural stimulation. Trace 2 represents the mathe-
matic sum of the responses from right and left ears. Trace 3 = [Trace 1 – Trace
2].

Permission was obtained for an electrocochleogram while she was in the operating room for a procedure not related to her ears. The electrocochleogram was expected to confirm what was thought to be simply peripheral deafness. However, extratympanic electrocochleography revealed responses in both ears down to 20 dB hearing level. Using the ABR technique, an aberrant dyssynchrony of the ABR was obtained after the second wave (Fig. 3). Subsequent ipsilateral reflex tests revealed normal ipsilateral reflexes but absent contralateral reflexes. This last observation implicated the IV ventricle structures.

Another example involves a child with a diagnosis of "autism." Behavioral audiometry, tympanometry, and reflexes suggested normal hearing, and yet the child ignored

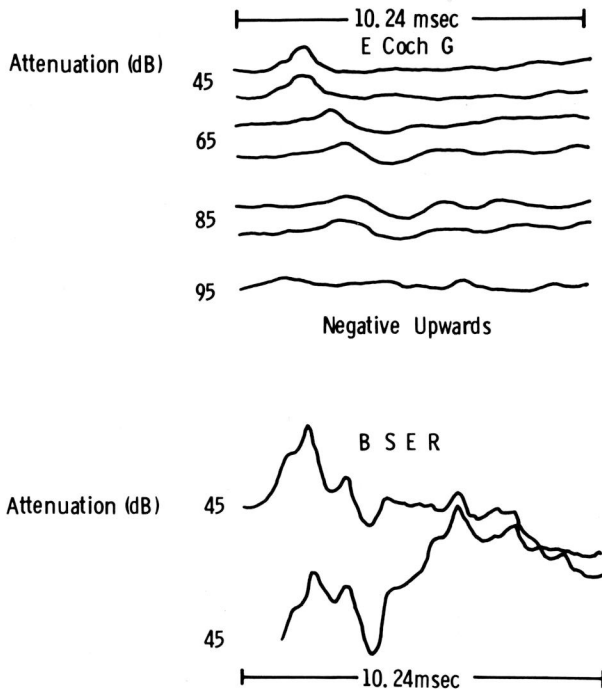

Fig. 3.   Normal electrocochleogram and aberrant ABR from "behaviorally unresponsive" child originally misdiagnosed as "deaf."

auditory stimulation and was essentially nonverbal. The ABR obtained using midline placement of the electrodes appeared abnormal, but most striking was the absence of the binaural-interaction response (Fig. 4).

A normal, binaural synchronous discharge could not be elicited during 2-ear stimulation. Animals which have had the IV ventricle bisected also fail to show this binaural interaction [25]. Although norms for children have not been established, norms for adults indicate that binaural interaction is readily measureable. Present data predicts that by 18 months, the normal ABR's latencies and magnitudes should be observed in human subjects.

SUMMARY

Although there has been some skepticism about the existence of central hearing loss because of the absence of an acceptable tool for its evaluation, techniques are now available for its measurement. There are some excellent behavioral methods available [1]. However, with judicious use of ABR, electrocochleography, and transcranially and ipsilaterally elicited middle-ear muscle reflexes, certain forms of central dysfunction can be studied physiologically.

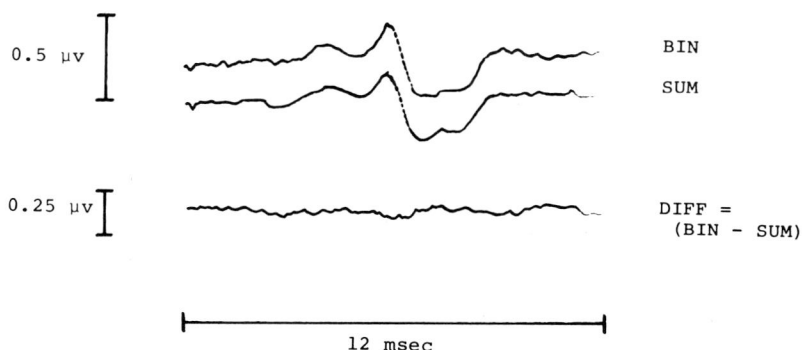

Fig. 4.   Absence of binaural interaction from a child with the diagnosis of autism.

REFERENCES

1. Jerger J, Jerger S: Clinical validity of central auditory tests. Scand Audiol 4:147, 1975.
2. Hodgson W: Audiological report of a patient with left hemispherectomy. J Speech Hear Disord 32:39, 1967.
3. Berlin CI, Lowe S: Temporal and dichotic factors in central auditory testing. In Katz J (ed): "Handbook of Clinical Audiology." Baltimore: Williams & Wilkins, 1972.
4. Hardy W: In Darley (ed): "Brain Mechanisms Underlying Speech and Language." New York: Grune and Stratton, 1967.
5. Berlin C, Wexler K, Jerger J, Halperin H, Smith S: Superior ultra-audiometric hearing: A new type of hearing loss which correlates highly with unusually good speech in the profoundly deaf. Otolaryngology 68:111, 1978.
6. Bordley J, Hardy W, Richter C: Audiometry with the use of the galvanic skin resistance response. Bull Johns Hopk Hosp 82:569, 1948.
7. Ventry I: Conditioned galvanic skin response audiometry. In Bradford L (ed): "Physiological Measures of the Audio-Vestibular System." New York: Academic Press, 1975.
8. Howe J, Miller CA: Midbrain deafness following head injury. Neurology 25:286, 1975.
9. Berlin C: New developments in evaluation of the central auditory mechanism. Ann Otol Rhinol Laryngol 85:833, 1976.
10. Webster D, Webster M: Effects of neonatal conductive hearing loss on brain stem auditory nuclei. Ann Otol Rhinol Laryngol 88:684, 1979.
11. Dobie R: Influence of otitis media on hearing and development. Ann Otol Rhinol Laryngol 88 (Suppl 60):48, 1979.
12. Landau W, Goldstein R, Kleffner F: Congenital aphasia: A clinicopathologic study. Neurology 10:915, 1960.
13. Jerger, J, Weikers N, Sharbrough FW, Jerger S: Bilateral lesions of the temporal lobe. Acta Otolaryngol (Suppl) 258, 1969.
14. Jewett D, Romano M, Williston J: Human auditory evoked potentials: Possible brain stem components detected on the scalp. Science 167:1517, 1970.
15. Jewett D, Williston J: Auditory-evoked far fields averaged from the scalp of humans. Brain 94:681, 1971.
16. Salamy A, McKean C, Buda F: Maturational changes in auditory transmission as reflected in human brain stem potentials. Brain Res 96:361, 1975.
17. Schulman-Galambos C, Galambos R: Brain stem auditory-evoked responses in premature infants. J Speech Hear Res 18:456, 1975.
18. Starr A, Achor J: Auditory brainstem response in neurological disease. Arch Neurol 32:761, 1975.
19. Martin M, Moore E: Scalp distribution of early (0-10 msec.) auditory evoked responses. Arch Otolaryngol 103:38, 1977.
20. Mokotoff B, Schulman-Galambos C, Galambos R: Brain stem auditory evoked responses in children. Arch Otolaryngol 103:38, 1977.
21. Dobie R, Berlin C: Binaural interaction in brainstem-evoked responses. Arch Otolaryngol 105:391, 1979.
22. Webster D, Webster M: Neonatal sound deprivation affects brain stem auditory nuclei. Arch Otolaryngol 103:392, 1977.

23. Rubel E, Rosenthal R: The ontogeny of auditory frequency generalization in the chicken. J Exp Psychol [Anim Behav] 1:287, 1975.
24. Clopton B, Winfield J: Effect of early exposure to patterned sound on unit activity in rat inferior colliculus. J Neurophysiol 39:1081, 1976.
25. Gardi J, Berlin C: Binaural interaction components of the guinea pig ABR: Possible origins. (Submitted for publication, Arch Otolaryngol 1979)

Hereditary Hearing Loss and Ear Dysplasia–Renal Adysplasia Syndromes: Syndrome Delineation and Possible Pathogenesis

Michael Melnick, DDS, PhD

Many malformation syndromes have external ear malformations as inconsistent features. However, other syndromes have external ear malformations as consistent and primary components of their phenotypes; these disorders may be divided into 3 groups: the otomandibular group, branchio-oto-dysplasia, and ear dysplasia–renal adysplasia [1]. The otomandibular group includes the so-called "1st and 2nd branchial arch syndrome" (oculoauriculovertebral dysplasia, hemifacial microsomia), mandibulofacial dysostosis (Treacher Collins syndrome), and the otomandibular dysostosis of Konigsmark and Gorlin [2]. The branchio-oto-dysplasia group includes patients with various external ear anomalies (such as preauricular tags, preauricular sinuses, and microtia) and branchial cleft anomalies (sinuses and fistulas), as well as conductive, sensorineural, or mixed hearing loss [3]. The ear dysplasia–renal adysplasia group includes syndromes with external ear malformations, branchial cleft anomalies, renal anomalies of various kinds, and hearing loss, primarily of a mixed or sensorineural type; these syndromes will be emphasized here. In addition to describing the syndromes in this group, the possible pathogenesis of the auricular and renal features of these syndromes will be presented.

EAR-KIDNEY ASSOCIATIONS

It has been observed for decades that nonsyndromic auricular malformations and renal malformations are as-

Birth Defects: Original Article Series, Volume XVI, Number 7, pages 59–72
© 1980 March of Dimes Birth Defects Foundation

sociated more frequently than one might expect [4]. In a recent study of nonsyndromic external ear anomalies [1], there was a group of patients with malformations of the urinary tract. This association may have been the result of chance, or may have occurred with greater frequency than could have been expected by chance alone. It was clear that the ear-kidney association was indeed a real association, since the relative risk of having any kidney anomaly was more than 3 times greater if the patient had an external ear anomaly; for a particular anomaly, atretic and/or double ureters, the relative risk was greater than 50 [1]. Whether these statistically significant associations can be classified as syndromes in their own right will not be argued here except to point out that the issue is probably moot.

EAR DYSPLASIA–RENAL ADYSPLASIA SYNDROMES

In 1957, Hilson published a report titled "Malformation of Ears as a Sign of Malformation of the Genito-Urinary Tract" [4]. In that report there were 4 relatively well-documented families:

Case 1: Proband (male, age 9) had severe lopping and cupping of the external ears and bilateral double ureters; father had identical anomalies; father's father and father's brother had similar ear anomalies and renal dysfunction, renal anomalies being suspected but unconfirmed; proband's brother had similar ear anomalies but an indeterminate pyelogram; the proband's other 2 brothers had normal ears and kidneys by pyelogram.

Case 2: Proband (male, age 4) had lopping and cupping of the external ears and bilateral double ureters; father had similar ear anomalies and kinking of the right ureter and bifid left renal pelvis; the father's mother, father's sister, and father's sister's son all had similar ear anomalies and renal dysfunction, renal anomalies being suspected but unconfirmed by pyelography; proband's brother was normal.

Case 3: Proband (male, newborn) had large, flat ears, typical "Potter facies," bilateral absence of kidneys, and hypospadias; father had left "bat-ear" and hypospadias;

father's mother had polycystic kidneys; although the father's sister was normal, she had 1 child with a single kidney, 2 children with left "bat-ears" and hypospadias but normal pyelograms, and 1 normal child.

Case 4: Proband (male, age 6) was described as having a "low-set deformed left ear" and a polycystic left kidney; father had a similar left ear and a polycystic left kidney; proband's brother had a cystic left kidney but normal ears; father's father and father's sister had malformed ears and polycystic kidneys.

It should be noted that all 4 pedigrees exhibited an autosomal dominant pattern of inheritance. Unfortunately, the results of audiometric testing were not reported for any of these families.

In 1961 Martins [5] reported another family with ear and renal anomalies. The proband, a 5-year-old male, had bilateral preauricular sinuses, bilateral branchial cleft sinuses, a hypoplastic right kidney, and a dilated left renal pelvis as well as absent superior calyces. The proband's mother and maternal grandmother both had bilateral preauricular and branchial cleft sinuses. Although an IVP was never done, it was noted that the proband's mother died at age 31 with a diagnosis of chronic nephritis. The results of audiologic studies were not noted for any members of this family. The pedigree suggests dominant inheritance, either autosomal or X-linked.

In 1968 Winter et al [6] described a family with autosomal recessive oto-renal-genital syndrome. Four female sibs had renal malformations, ranging from unilateral hypoplasia to bilateral absence of kidneys, vaginal atresia, low-set and lop ears, atresia of the external auditory meatus, varying anomalies of the middle ear ossicles, and conductive hearing loss.

Recently, Melnick et al [7, 8] reported a family with a syndrome designated autosomal dominant branchio-oto-renal dysplasia (BOR syndrome). Their report described a 2-generation family of 9 individuals in which the father and 3 of the 6 living children all had: 1) a mixed hearing loss with a Mondini cochlear malformation and stapes fixation; 2) cup-shaped, anteverted pinnae with bilateral preauricular sinuses; 3) bilateral branchial cleft fistulas; 4) kidney hypoplasia and dysplasia, including dysplastic calyces. A 4th child, who died at 5 months of age, was reported at autopsy to have branchial cleft fistulas and bilateral polycystic kidneys. Subsequently, several reports of families with similar anomalies have been reported [3, 9, 10]. The branchial anomalies have been variable: lop ears, cup ears, hypoplastic ears, preauricular sinuses, branchial cleft sinuses, ear lobe sinuses, and various dysplasias of the middle ear ossicles. The renal anomalies also have been variable: kidney agenesis/aplasia, kidney hypoplasia, polycystic kidneys, calyceal dysplasia, bifid renal pelvis, and bifid ureters. Based on the families reported to date [3, 7-10], there is usually a major sensorineural component to the hearing loss with cochlear dysplasia, usually of the Mondini type.

The 2 sons in the family with BOR dysplasia reported by Melnick et al [3] and the daughter in the report by Fitch and Srolovitz [9] raise an important diagnostic consideration: in addition to true auricular *malformation,* they have a pattern of anomalies characteristic of the "Potter syndrome." Buchta et al [11] have designated this syndromic entity as a "symptomatic deformity complex" consisting of malformations (micrognathia, pulmonary hypoplasia, ureto-bladder anomalies, and occasionally cleft palate) and deformations (flat nose, large, flat auricles, talipes equinovarus, and other limb anomalies) both of which are associated with oligohydramnios. Oligohydramnios may result from bilateral renal agenesis or severe dysplasia, or from other causes of decreased amniotic fluid [12]. True auricular dysmorphogenesis, as described in the family with BOR dysplasia by Melnick et al [3], Fitch and Srolovitz [9], and case 3 of the Hilson report [4], is most often present in cases of renal agenesis associated with true multiple congenital anomaly syndromes [11]. These syndromes have been grouped by Buchta et al [11] into a genetically heterogeneous category called "hereditary renal adysplasia" (HRA): adysplasia is a composite term for agenesis and dysplasia and implies predominantly asymmetric involvement or, less commonly, bilateral agenesis or symmetric dysplasia.

Syndromes which would fall in the subcategory of HRA with ear malformations include the BOR syndrome [3, 4 (Hilson cases 1 and 2), 5, 7-10], the dysmorphic pinna-hypospadias-renal adysplasia syndrome [4(Hilson case 3)], the dysmorphic pinna-polycystic kidney syndrome [4(Hilson case 4)], and probably the oto-renal-genital syndrome of Winter et al [6]. The first 3 syndromes are autosomal dominant and have many overlapping features; it is not known whether they represent the same entity, multiple alleles, or multiple loci. The oto-renal-genital syndrome is most likely autosomal recessive.

POSSIBLE PATHOGENESIS OF EXTERNAL AND MIDDLE EAR MALFORMATIONS

By the 28th day of embryonic life 4 well-developed pairs of branchial arches are visible (Fig. 1). The external ear is derived from the ectoderm and mesenchyme of the 1st (mandibular) and 2nd (hyoid) branchial arches. The middle ear ossicles are derived from the cartilages in these arches—the Meckel cartilage (1st arch) giving rise to the incus and malleus and the Reichert cartilage (2nd arch) giving rise to the stapes. The most critical period of development for the external and middle ear is between the 5th and 8th week of embryonic life.

At about day 38 the smooth margins of the 1st and 2nd arches begin to develop small swellings or hillocks. Three hillocks appear on the caudal border of the mandibular arch and 3 on the cephalic border of the 2nd arch (Fig. 2). These swellings are the result of mesenchymal cell proliferation. By day 41 the hillocks have reached their maximum size, have moved in a more dorsal and lateral direction and have begun to fuse. Fusion is complete by the 43rd–45th day of embryonic life (Fig. 3). At this time the amount of mesenchyme in each of the 1st and 2nd arches is about equal. However, from the end of the 7th week or the beginning of the 8th, through subsequent fetal development, the amount of 2nd arch mesenchyme substantially increases relative to 1st arch mesenchyme. By the 20th week of development the ear is nearly ana-

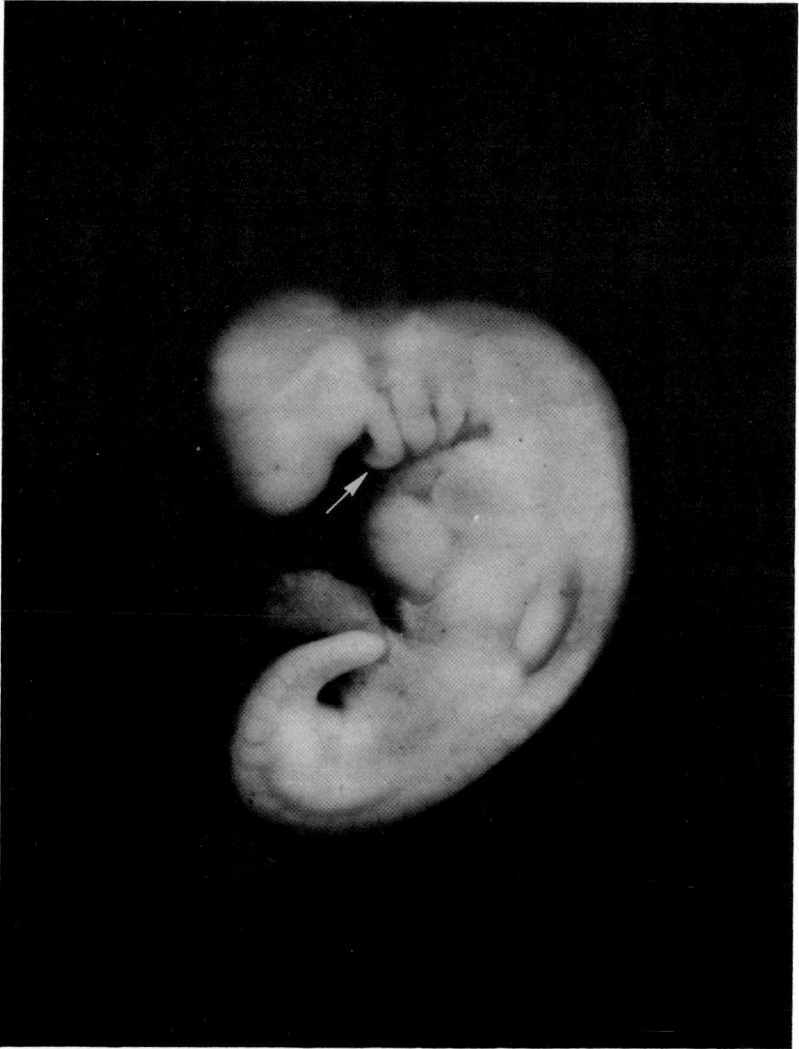

Fig. 1. Lateral view of human embryo at Carnegie stage 13 (length: 4-6 mm age: circa 28 days). Note the presence of 4 well-defined branchial arches (arrow), designated from left to right as I (mandibular), II (hyoid), III, and IV. Figs. 1–4 courtesy of Professor Hideo Nishimura, Central Institute for Experimental Animals, Kawasaki, Japan.)

tomically complete. The only portions of the ear derived from the 1st arch are the tragus and possibly the anterior crus of the helix margin, while the 2nd arch derivatives include the helix, anthelix, scapha, antitragus, and the lobule.

The dorsal end of the 1st branchial cleft (between arches I and II) is beginning to widen while the auricle is developing (Figs. 2 and 3) and becomes a distinct structure termed the fossa angularis. The ectodermal cells at the bottom of this fossa proliferate and expand inward as a solid core known as the meatal plug. By the 70th day of development this plug begins to approach the expanding tympanic cavity and its central cells are degenerating to form a cavity which ultimately becomes the external auditory meatus.

Clearly, normal development of external and middle ear structures is dependent on the integrity of the early development of the 1st and 2nd branchial arches. For example, hypoplasia of the 1st and/or 2nd arches (Fig. 4) results in dysplasias of structures derived from them such as the upper lip, mandible, external ear, and middle ear [13]. The quality and quantity of arch abnormality will determine the subsequent anatomic malformations in the newborn.

Faulty development later in embryonic life also results in ear malformation. Failure of the auricular hillocks to develop through mesenchymal proliferation will result in either anotia or microtia. Lop, cup, and protruding ears probably represent faulty differentiation (dysplasia) of the 2nd arch hillocks, but to a degree considerably less than microtia. It has generally been assumed that preauricular sinuses result from incomplete fusion of the 1st arch hillocks. However, since the sinuses are not necessarily at points of fusion, this explanation is not satisfactory. Some investigators have suggested that the sinuses may be related to defective closure of the most dorsal part of the 1st branchial cleft [14], while others indicate that they represent ectodermal folds that are sequestered during auricle formation [15]. Preauricular tags are thought to result from the development of accessory auricular hillocks [14]. Finally, atresia of the external auditory meatus results from a failure of the meatal plug to canalize [14].

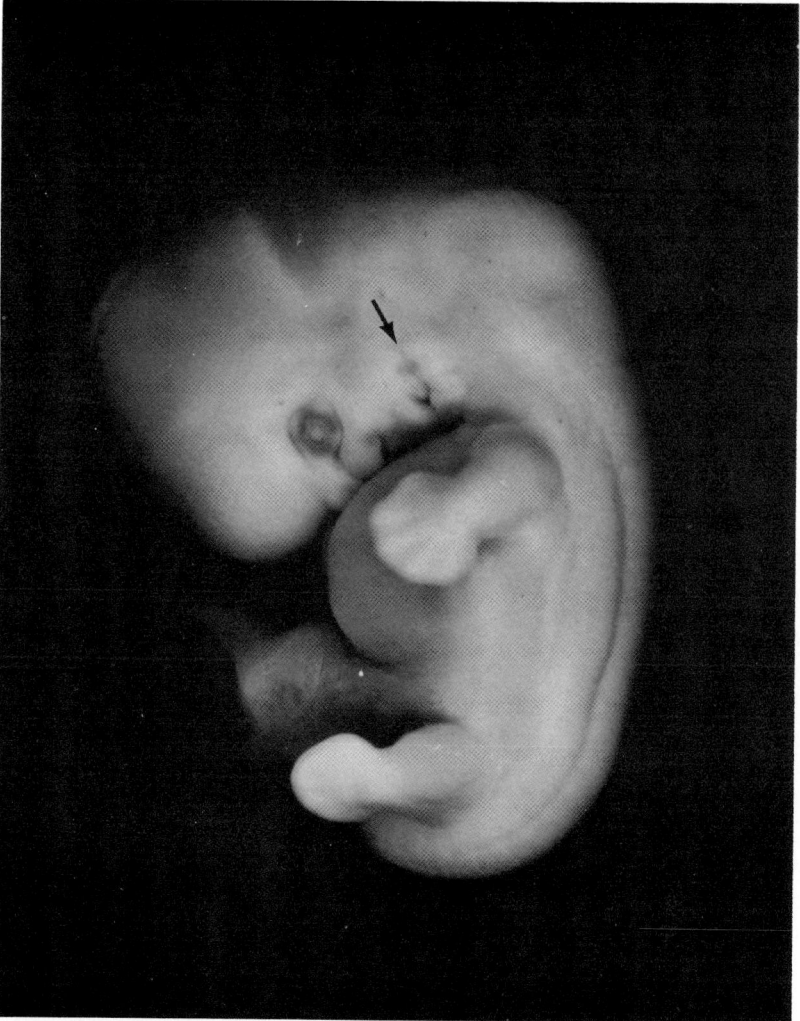

Fig. 2.   Lateral view of human embryo at Carnegie stage 18 (length: 13-17 mm; age: circa 44 days). The arrow points to the 6 auricular hillocks which have begun to fuse on either side of the 1st branchial cleft.

Abnormalities of the incus and malleus are most often due to incomplete or atypical differentiation of the dorsal end of the Meckel (1st arch) cartilage. This dysplasia is seen as malformed individual ossicles, bony union of 2 otherwise normally formed ossicles, or fusion of 2 mal-

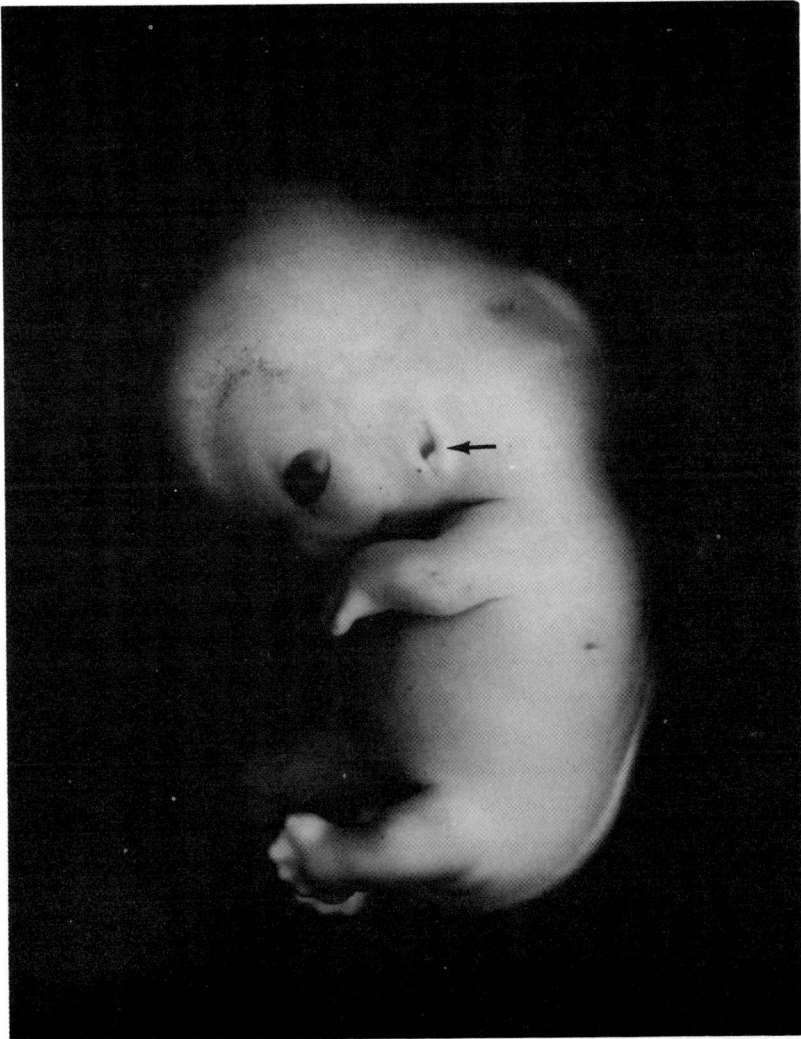

Fig. 3. Lateral view of human embryo at Carnegie stage 20 (length: 18-22 mm; age: circa 50.5 days). Note that the fused hillocks have continued to develop into a recognizable rudimentary pinna (arrow).

formed ossicles. Failure of differentiation (dysplasia) of the fibrous annular ligament attached to the footplate of the stapes results in bony fixation of the stapes to the otic capsule [14].

It has been assumed by some investigators that each of

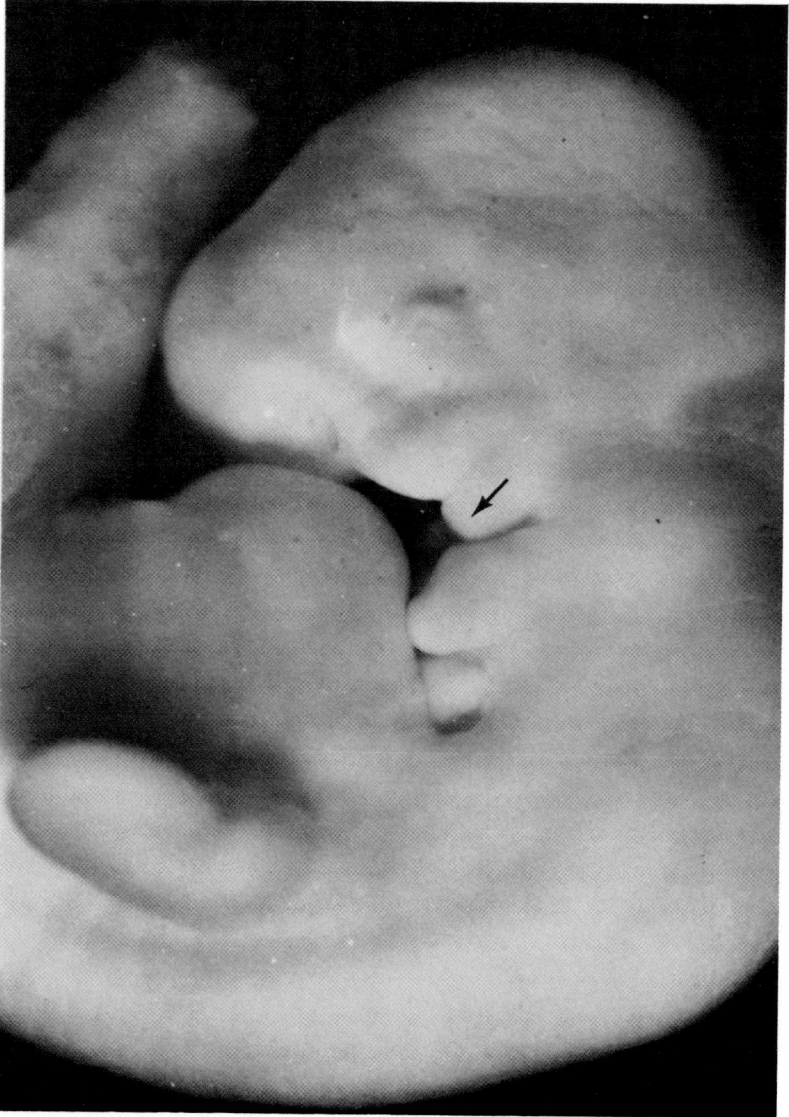

Fig. 4. Lateral view of human embryo at Carnegie stage 16 (length: 8-11mm; circa 37 days). Note the hypoplasia of branchial arch I (arrow).

these external ear anomalies has a distinct etiology [16]. This, however, may not be so with all cases. The ear malformations in the syndromes discussed above are variable among and within families with the same syndrome, and may even be different between sides in the same person [3]. Furthermore, in a large prospective study of nonsyndromic external ear malformations, it was found that many types of ear anomalies in a single individual are more likely associated with multiple hits by a single etiology; thus, any ear malformation of the type mentioned above is not necessarily etiologically distinct from any other type [1].

POSSIBLE PATHOGENESIS OF THE RENAL ANOMALIES

As with the external and middle ear, the most critical period for renal development is between the 5th and 8th weeks. The metanephros ("permanent kidney") begins to develop early in the 5th week from 2 embryonic structures: the ureteric bud and the metanephrogenic mesodermal mass [14]. The ureteric bud arises from the mesonephric duct near its entry into the cloaca, and gives rise to the ureter, renal pelvis, major and minor calyces, and collecting tubules. The bud grows in a dorsocranial direction into the metanephrogenic mass, which forms a mesodermal cap over the ureteric bud. The stalk of the ureteric bud becomes the ureter; the expanded cranial end of the bud forms the renal pelvis, which then divides into major and minor calyces; and the collecting tubules grow from the minor calyces. Each collecting tubule undergoes repeated branching to form successive generations of collecting tubules. Near the blind end of each arched collecting tubule, clusters of mesenchymal cells develop into metanephric tubules. Differentiation of the metanephric tubules depends upon an inductive stimulus from the ureteric bud and its derivatives [14, 17]. The renal corpuscle and its associated tubules form a nephron. The distal convoluted tubule of the nephron contacts an arched collecting tubule, and the 2 tubules become confluent. Embryologically, a uriniferous tubule consists of the secretory tubule of the nephron derived from the metanephrogenic mass and a collecting tubule from the ureteric bud [14].

The renal anomalies in the syndromes described above

can all be explained as variable failures of ureteric bud differentiation. These failures can be thought of as a progressive continuum:

absence of ureteric bud	→	renal agenesis
failure of ureteric bud to grow	→	renal aplasia
generalized hypoplasia of ureteric bud	→	hypoplastic kidney
precocious division of ureteric bud	→	bifid ureters or pelvis
incomplete or failed end-stage division of ureteric bud	→	dysplasias of calyces and/or collecting tubules

Polycystic kidneys may represent failure of many nephrons derived from the metanephrogenic mass to join with the collecting tubules derived from the ureteric bud, the primary dysplasia being a failure of collecting tubule differentiation. In summary, the common denominator of all these anomalies could rest with the variable ability of the ureteric bud to grow and divide into its required component parts.

CONCLUSION

Auricular malformation, hearing loss, and renal adysplasia are sometimes associated as features of multiple congenital anomaly syndromes. These syndromes can be grouped into a genetically heterogeneous category termed "hereditary ear dysplasia — renal adysplasia syndromes." Syndromes in this category include branchio-oto-renal adysplasia, dysmorphic pinna — hypospadias — renal adysplasia syndrome, dysmorphic pinna — polycystic kidney syndrome, and oto-renal-genital (Winter) syndrome. The first 3 syndromes are autosomal dominant but have features in common; the last syndrome is autosomal recessive. The pathogenesis of the ear anomalies appears to include variable degrees of failed branchial arch and/or auricular hillock growth and development, while the pathogenesis of the renal anomalies could include variable degrees of failed ureteric bud growth and development. These events raise the interesting possibility that the pleiotropic manifestation of these mutant genes is related to cell division in embryologically disparate structures.

Audiologic assessment of patients with these syndromes is well characterized only for branchio-oto-renal dysplasia and oto-renal-genital syndrome. In the former, there is almost always a major sensorineural component to the hearing loss with varying degrees of cochlear dysplasia, notably of the Mondini type. The hearing loss in oto-renal-genital syndrome is thus far exclusively of the conductive type with various kinds of ossicular fixation and atresia of the external auditory meatus.

It is imperative that both audiologic *and* renal studies be performed in all patients with familial branchial arch malformations, because of the clinical implications of an unrecognized prelingual hearing loss and the prognostic importance for genetic counseling if renal malformations are found. Similarly, the parents and sibs of infants with "Potter facies" in the presence of auricular *malformation* and renal adysplasia should be evaluated for evidence of branchial arch malformation, hearing loss, or renal anomalies in order to rule out a hereditary ear dysplasia–renal adysplasia syndrome.

REFERENCES

1. Melnick M, Myrianthopoulos NC: "External Ear Malformations: Epidemiology, Genetics, and Natural History." New York: Alan R Liss for the March of Dimes Birth Defects Foundation, BD:OAS XV(9), 1979.
2. Konigsmark BW, Gorlin RJ: "Genetic and Metabolic Deafness." Philadelphia: WB Saunders, 1976.
3. Melnick M, Hodes ME, Nance WE, Yune H, Sweeney A: Branchio-oto-renal dysplasia and branchio-oto dysplasia: Two distinct autosomal dominant disorders. Clin Genet 13:425–442, 1978.
4. Hilson D: Malformations of ears as a sign of malformation of the genitourinary tract. Br Med J 2:785–789, 1957.
5. Martins AG: Lateral cervical and preauricular sinuses: Their transmission as dominant characters. Br Med J 2:255–256, 1961.
6. Winter JSD, Kohn G, Mellman WJ, Wagner S: A familial syndrome of renal, genital and middle ear anomalies. J Pediatr 72:88–93, 1968.
7. Melnick M, Bixler D, Silk K, Yune H, Nance WE: Autosomal dominant branchio-otorenal dysplasia. In Bergsma D (ed): "New Chromosomal and

Malformation Syndromes." Miami:Symposia Specialists for The National Foundation-March of Dimes, BD:OAS XI(5):121–128, 1975.

8. Melnick M, Bixler D, Nance WE, Silk K, Yune H: Familial branchio-oto-renal dysplasia: A new addition to the branchial arch syndromes. Clin Genet 9:25–34, 1976.

9. Fitch N, Srolovitz H: Severe renal dysgenesis produced by a dominant gene. Am J Dis Child 130:1356–1357, 1976.

10. Fraser FC, Ling D, Clogg D, Nogrady B: Genetic aspects of the BOR syndrome—Branchial fistulas, ear pits, hearing loss, and renal anomalies. Am J Med Genet 2:241–252, 1978.

11. Buchta R, Viseskul C, Gilbert EF, Santo GE, Opitz JM: Familial bilateral renal agenesis and hereditary renal adysplasia. Z Kinderheilkd 115:111–129, 1973.

12. Barr M, Burdi AR: Potter syndrome with and without fetal renal abnormality. Teratology 13:16A, 1976.

13. Nashimura H, Okamato N: "Sequential Atlas of the Human Congenital Malformations." Baltimore:University Park Press, 1976, pp 76–83.

14. Moore KL: "The Developing Human: Clinically Oriented Embryology." Philadelphia: WB Saunders, 1973.

15. Aronsohn RS, Batsakis JG, Rice DH, Work WP: Anomalies of the first branchial cleft. Arch Otolaryngol 102:737–740, 1976.

16. McKusick VA: "Mendelian Inheritance in Man. Catalogs of Autosomal Dominant, Autosomal Recessive, and X-Linked Phenotypes," 5th Ed. Baltimore: The Johns Hopkins University Press, 1978.

17. Gluecksohn-Waelsch S: Genetic control of mammalian differentiation. In "Genetics Today," vol. 2, Proc XI Internat Congr Genetics. The Hague, Netherlands, 1963.

Hereditary Hearing Loss Associated With Musculoskeletal Malformations

Robert J. Gorlin, DDS, MS

More than 30 genetic musculoskeletal disorders that have greater than chance association with hearing loss are known. Because of obvious constraints, it is only possible to discuss a few here. Each disorder has been discussed in detail elsewhere [1]; therefore, only the salient features of each condition will be described.

OTOPALATODIGITAL SYNDROME

The otopalatodigital (OPD) syndrome is characterized by conductive hearing loss, cleft palate, pugilistic facies, generalized bone dysplasia, and growth retardation. Since the first description by Dudding et al [2], several large kindreds have been studied. Two of the best radiologic studies are those of Poznanski et al [3], and Kozlowski et al [4].

The facies is characterized by an overhanging brow with large supraorbital ridges, flat midface, antimongoloid obliquity of palpebral fissures, ocular hypertelorism, and broad flat nasal bridge (Fig. 1). The terminal phalanges are wide and the halluces abbreviated. The toes are broad and variably curved; frequently there is webbing between the toes. Mild mental retardation is frequent.

A bilateral 30–90 dB conductive hearing loss has been noted on audiometric testing. On tympanotomy, thickened and malformed ossicles have been found [1]. The most prominent radiographic findings include an almost vertical clivus, frequent posterior dislocation of the radial heads, and oar-shaped 2nd and 3rd metatarsals.

The syndrome is transmitted in an X-linked manner, female heterozygotes having prominent lateral supraorbital ridges and minor skeletal alterations [3,5].

Birth Defects: Original Article Series, Volume XVI, Number 7, pages 73—87
© 1980 March of Dimes Birth Defects Foundation

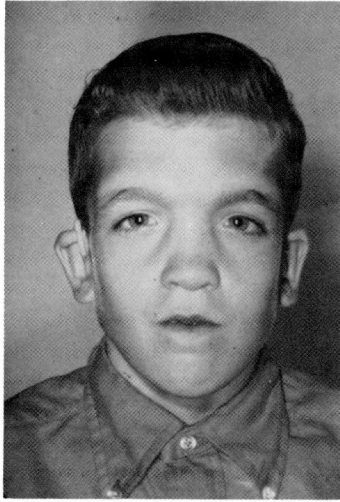

Fig. 1. Otopalatodigital syndrome: Overhanging brow with prominent supraorbital ridges and wide nasal bridge gives pugilistic appearance.

DOMINANT CRANIOMETAPHYSEAL DYSPLASIA

Craniometaphyseal dysplasia is characterized by hyperostosis of the cranial and facial bones and splaying of the metaphyseal ends of long bones [6]. Inheritance of craniometaphyseal dysplasia is clearly autosomal dominant with marked variability in expression [7]. The earlier literature has erroneously designated this disorder as Pyle disease, a disorder which is inherited as an autosomal recessive.

Usually, within the first year of life, the root of the nose begins to broaden [8]. Increasing bony hyperostosis often narrows the nasal lumen, leading to obstruction and open mouth (Fig. 2A). There may be visual loss due to optic atrophy. Facial nerve paralysis, headache, or vertigo occur in at least one-third of patients. Some patients have complained of facial paresthesia. Hearing loss, noted in about half the patients, begins in childhood and is slowly progressive until, by the 3rd or 4th decade, there is a 30–90 dB loss. The loss is largely conductive,

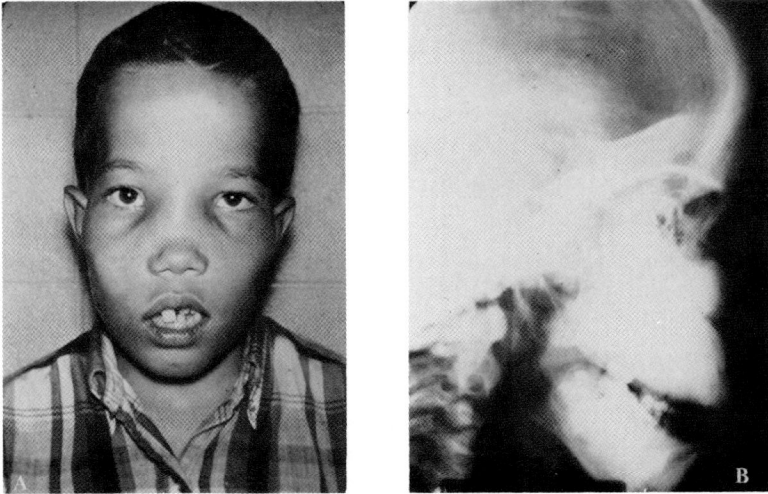

Fig. 2. Dominant craniometaphyseal dysplasia: A) Note widened nasal bridge. B) Note frontal hyperostosis, sclerosis of skull base and facial bones, under-pneumatization of sinuses and mastoids.

although in several cases there has been a sensorineural component. Vestibular tests have been normal [9].

On radiographs, the calvaria exhibits frontal and occipital hyperostosis and sclerosis (Fig. 2B). The paranasal sinuses and mastoids may be obliterated or nonpneumatized. The long bones have a club-shaped metaphyseal flare; associated with the flare is diaphyseal sclerosis which disappears with age.

RECESSIVE CRANIOMETAPHYSEAL DYSPLASIA

This disorder is clinically and pathologically more severe than dominant craniometaphyseal dysplasia. Marked ocular hypertelorism is a constant feature, and blindness due to optic atrophy has been described in several cases. Facial paresis has also been reported in most patients. Hearing loss is as severe as that found in the dominant form.

Hyperostosis of the calvaria with widening of the cranial cortex, sclerosis of the skull base, ocular hypertelorism, and absent paranasal sinuses have been noted in all patients. Long bone changes may be more severe than those seen in the dominant form. Due to insufficient documentation of supposedly recessive cases and the extreme variability of expression in the dominant form of the disorder, more well-studied patients are needed to determine the existence of recessive craniometaphyseal dysplasia [6, 10–12].

CRANIODIAPHYSEAL DYSPLASIA

Craniodiaphyseal dysplasia is a term coined by Gorlin et al [6] to designate an autosomal recessive bone disorder characterized by massive generalized hyperostosis and sclerosis primarily involving the skull and facial bones, which are severely thickened, distorted, and enlarged [13–16]. The first signs of the disorder are nasal obstruction and recurrent upper respiratory infections during the first few years, or even during the first few months of life, followed by marked bony thickening, ocular hypertelorism, nasal flattening, and severe dental malocclusion. Bilateral choanal stenosis occurs causing the patient to keep the mouth open to breathe (Fig. 3). Growth is retarded and early death is common. All patients have severe ocular hypertelorism, lacrimal duct obstruction, and diminished visual acuity or blindness due to optic atrophy. Cranial nerves are compressed. Developmental milestones are delayed and there is progressive mental retardation, headache, and seizures. Lack of sexual maturity is common.

Severe hearing impairment has been noted in all cases. In most cases, the loss has been mixed. On radiographs, the skull and facial bones as well as the mandible are severely sclerotic and hyperostotic. The paranasal sinuses and mastoids do not develop. The ribs and clavicles are thickened and sclerotic. The long tubular bones do not have metaphyseal flare, but rather the shape of a policeman's nightstick; diaphyseal endostosis is noted. The short tubular bones of the hands and feet, especially the

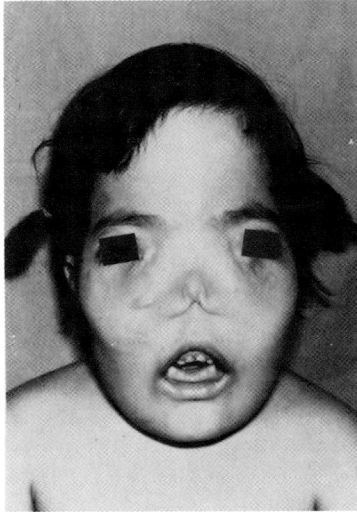

Fig. 3. Craniodiaphyseal dysplasia: Five-year-old patient showing marked enlargement of cranium, facial bones, and mandible. Note severe ocular hypertelorism and dental malocclusion. (From Macpherson RI: Craniodiaphyseal dysplasia, a disease or group of diseases. J Can Assoc Radiol 25:22–23, 1974, with permission.)

1st metatarsal, are cylindric. Serum alkaline phosphatase levels may be elevated during the active phase of the disorder.

FRONTOMETAPHYSEAL DYSPLASIA

Since the original definition of frontometaphyseal dysplasia by Gorlin and Cohen [17], at least a dozen additional pedigrees have been published [18–23]. Initially, the mode of inheritance was controversial and genetic heterogeneity was suspected. However, Gorlin and Winter [24] have demonstrated that the disorder is X-linked.

The marked supraorbital ridges, wide nasal bridge, and small pointed chin are striking (Fig. 4A). There is progressive wasting of muscles of the arms and legs, especially the hypothenar and interosseous muscles of the hands. Dorsiflexion of the wrists and extension of the elbows are reduced; pronation and supination become

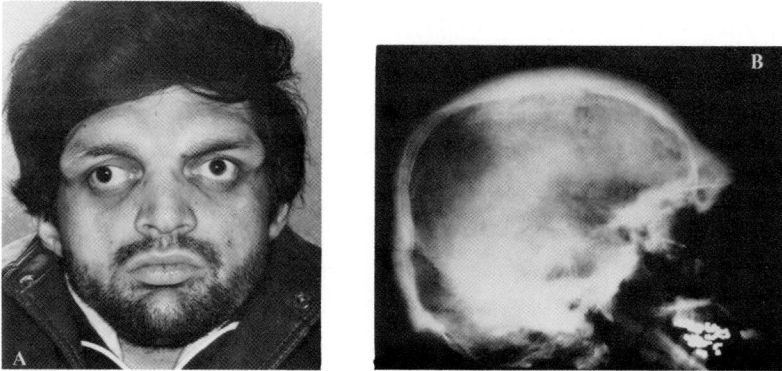

Fig. 4. Frontometaphyseal dysplasia: A) Marked supraorbital ridge, wide nasal bridge, and exotropia give this 32-year-old male patient a striking appearance. B) Radiograph of skull showing supraorbital torus, hypoplasia and dysplasia of mandible.

extremely limited. Missing permanent teeth and retained deciduous teeth have been noted in several reports.

Most patients have moderate conductive hearing loss, although in some cases symmetric progressive mixed hearing loss has been described; fixation of the malleus to the incus has been noted.

On radiographs, there is a thick, torus-like frontal ridge; the frontal sinuses are absent (Fig. 4B). Prominent antegonial notching with marked hypoplasia of the angle and coronoid process has been documented. The diaphyseal regions of the long bones are more dense than normal, and the metaphyseal areas lack normal modeling; an Erlenmeyer flask deformity is thus produced. There is marked flaring of the iliac bones, widened elongated middle phalanges, slender ribs, and increased interpediculate distances in the lumbar spine.

RECESSIVE OSTEOPETROSIS (ALBERS-SCHÖNBERG DISEASE)

Osteopetrosis or marble-bone disease is genetically heterogeneous [25]. Hearing loss as a consistent finding has been reported only in recessive osteopetrosis [26,27]. Increased density of all bones due to failure of absorption

of the primary spongiosa results in anemia, hepatospleno-
megaly, thrombocytopenia, blindness, hearing loss, facial
palsy, and osteomyelitis. The disorder can be recognized
at birth or even in utero. Death usually results within the
first few years of life from anemia or secondary infection,
although there have been recent attempts to use bone
marrow transplants. To date, none has met with success.

The head is enlarged and may exhibit frontal and parie-
tal bossing. There also may be mild ocular hypertelorism.
Growth is retarded in about a third of the cases. Osteomyelitis of the jaws occurs in about 20% of the cases as a
complication of dental extraction, presumably due to defi-
cient blood supply. Fractures have been noted in about a
third of the cases. Visual loss is seen in over 80% of
these infants, and begins in the first year of life; the loss
may result from retinal atrophy rather than from optic
atrophy secondary to pressure on the optic nerve. Unilateral or bilateral facial palsy occurs during the first few
years of life in only about 10% of patients, probably
secondary to pressure of the dense bone of the internal
acoustic meatus on the VIIth cranial nerve. In about half
the patients there is enlargement of the liver and spleen
because of the extramedullary hemopoiesis. Between
25% and 50% of the patients who do not die within the
first few years of life have moderate mixed hearing loss
beginning in childhood; in about half of the cases there is
a history of otitis media.

DOMINANT SYMPHALANGISM AND CONDUCTIVE HEARING LOSS

Conductive deafness due to fixation of the stapedial
footplate in combination with absence of the proximal
and interphalangeal joints and carpotarsal bone coalition
has been described in many kindreds as an autosomal
dominant condition [28–30]. For unknown reasons, the
disorder has been mistakenly called Nievergelt-Pearlman
syndrome [31], a different disorder.

Little or no movement is possible in the proximal interphalangeal joints of the fingers, usually from birth (Fig.
5A). The skin over the affected joints is shiny and usually

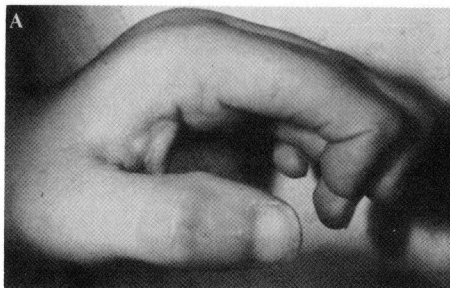

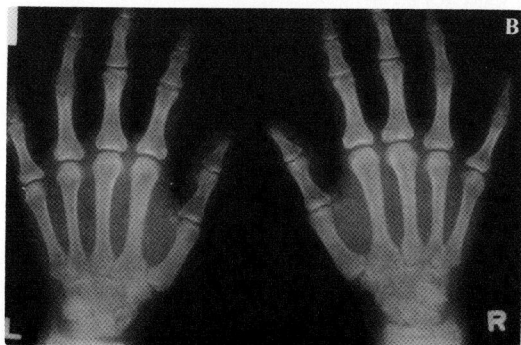

Fig. 5. Dominant symphalangism and conduction deafness: A) Proximal symphalangism prevents normal closure of the hand; fingers not all affected to same degree. B) Radiograph of patient showing mild radial deviation of 3rd through 5th digits; 2 phalanges in 4th and 5th digits are the result of fusion. Note fusion of lesser multangular and capitate, and triquetral with hamate. (From Gorlin RJ et al: Stapes fixation and proximal symphalangism. Z Kinderheilkd 108:12–16, 1970, with permission.)

lacks hairs or wrinkles. When several fingers are involved, all digits ulnar to the most radially affected digit have the same fusion anomaly. Neither the thumb nor the metacarpophalangeal joints are involved. The feet often have a prominence on the medial side of the distal end of the navicular bone and there is usually another prominence at the base of the 5th metatarsal. Tarsal coalition results in decreased movement at the subtalar and submetatarsal joints. The feet are usually flat and the ankles broad. The ability to invert and evert the foot is reduced. Occasionally, the patient may walk on the external border of the feet or, rarely, on the toes.

Bilateral conductive hearing loss is variable in degree among patients. Bony fusion between the stapes and the petrous portion of the temporal bone has been noted on tympanotomy. By adolescence, there is complete bony fusion of the proximal interphalangeal joints of the little finger; less commonly, fusion of the joints in the other fingers is evident. Anomalies of the carpal bones include malsegmentation of the triquetrum, and partial fusion of the triquetrum to both the lunate and hamate (Fig. 5B). Talonavicular fusion is usually found.

MULTIPLE SYNOSTOSES AND CONDUCTIVE HEARING LOSS: SYMPHALANGISM-BRACHYDACTYLY SYNDROME

Maroteaux et al [32] and Herrmann [33] reported kindreds with multiple synostoses and conductive hearing loss, and I have seen an isolated case. The facies may be unusual, the nose being long and thin with minimal alar flare. The patient may walk with a waddling gait, on the outer border of the feet, without resting on the heels. The upper arms are short. Often, there is cubitus valgus with dislocation of the head of the radius and limitation of pronation, supination, and extension of the elbow. The fingers are short. All proximal interphalangeal finger joints lack skin creases. Fingernails or toenails may be hypoplastic and the terminal portions of the fingers and toes may be missing. Proximal metacarpals and metatarsals are rarely absent.

Conductive hearing loss appearing during early childhood or adolescence was noted in 4 of 6 patients reported by Herrmann [33] and in 4 of 7 patients reported by Maroteaux et al [32]. Complete ankylosis of the stapes was noted on tympanotomy. Inheritance is autosomal dominant.

Char [34] described a child with sensorineural hearing loss associated with brachydactyly. There were 2 phalanges in each digit; there were no fingernails or toenails.

SCLEROSTEOSIS (VAN BUCHEM DISEASE)

Initially believed to be 2 different disorders, sclerosteosis and van Buchem disease are, in my opinion, the

same. The disorder is characterized by generalized os-
teosclerosis and hyperostosis with syndactyly of the digits. Hirsch [35] may have been the first to report the
condition. Seven cases were reported by van Buchem et
al [36] in 1962 to which he added another 8 patients in
1971 [37]. The many reports of the disorder have been
reviewed by Konigsmark and Gorlin [1, pp 169–174]. An
additional 25 affected individuals in 15 kindreds in South
Africa were described by Beighton et al [38]. The disorder is inherited as an autosomal recessive.

The typical facies develops early in childhood, but
becomes progressively more severe with age. It is characterized by a steep high forehead, ocular hypertelorism,
broad flat nasal root, midface hypoplasia, and a prognathic, broad, square mandible. Often there is exophthalmos
(Fig. 6). Head circumference is enlarged and body height
is increased. Many of the patients reported by Beighton
et al [38] had asymmetric cutaneous syndactyly of the
index and middle fingers. Rarely, mild syndactyly may
involve and 3rd and 4th fingers. The nails of involved
fingers are frequently dysplastic.

Facial nerve paralysis may be congenital, but more
frequently it appears in infancy or childhood. Initially, it
is usually unilateral, but becomes bilateral in late adolescence. Chronic headache and decreased sensory function
of the 1st and 2nd divisions of the trigeminal nerve are
common findings. Anosmia has also been described. In
early adult life there may be unilateral or bilateral
compression of the optic nerves, papilledema, optic atrophy, and reduced visual fields. Bilateral sensorineural,
mixed, or conductive hearing loss, a constant feature of
the disorder, may appear early in infancy, during childhood, or late in adolescence.

On radiographs, the calvaria is greatly thickened and
dense, and its inner and outer tables become unrecogniz-
able. The cranial base is especially thickened. The body
of the mandible is greatly enlarged and prognathic, and
the angle is more obtuse than normal. The rami are only
minimally involved. The clavicles and ribs are broadened
as a result of cortical thickening. The scapulae, pelvis,

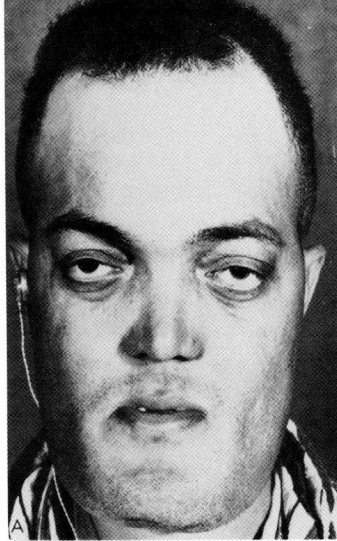

Fig. 6. Sclerosteosis: Marked mandibular growth following puberty; mandible assumes square form. Mixed deafness, facial palsy, headache, exophthalmos, and blindness are common complications (Courtesy of CJ Witkop, Jr, Minneapolis, Minnesota.)

and vertebral bodies are uniformly sclerotic. The tubular bones are more dense than normal and lack diaphyseal modeling. The middle phalanx of the index finger may be small and triangular, or absent.

Serum alkaline phosphatase levels are markedly elevated in nearly all patients.

KNIEST DYSPLASIA

In 1952 Kniest [39] described a rare form of disproportionate dwarfism. Inheritance is autosomal dominant [40–42]. Patients with this disorder have a round face and depressed nasal bridge. The neck is short and the head appears to sit upon the thorax. Cleft palate, shortened limbs, clubfeet, and prominent knees are frequently noted at birth. Lumbar lordosis with dorsal kyphosis usually develops within the first few years of life, resulting in reduced height of the trunk. The child may not sit until 2 years of age, and may not begin to walk until 3 years. By the 4th year of life most joints have become enlarged, stiff and painful, especially those of the knees, elbows, and wrists. Flexion and extension of most joints become progressively reduced. The gait is waddling. Thoracic scoliosis may develop later in the course of the disease [43].

Myopia of greater than 10 diopters have been present in about 50% of published cases. Conductive hearing loss has been described by a number of authors [40, 44].

On radiographs of infants with the disorder, the long bones are short and have enlarged metaphyses. The metaphyses of long bones flare and the epiphyses around the knees are large, irregular, and radiolucent. In childhood, the distal ends of the proximal phalanges of the fingers have pseudoepiphyses. The proximal row of carpal bones is usually small. The iliac wings are broad and reduced in height, especially in relation to the large capital femoral epiphysis and proximal femoral metaphysis. Usually there is coxa vara. The vertebral height is reduced and there is anterior wedging of vertebral bodies.

AUTOSOMAL RECESSIVE HYPERPHOSPHATASIA

Autosomal recessive hyperphosphatasia, or juvenile Paget disease, has many names (hyperostosis corticalis deformans juvenilis, familial osteoectasia with macrocranium, osteochalasia desmalis familiaris, etc) [45–49]. It is characterized by progressive skeletal deformities that become apparent during the 2nd or 3rd year of life and result in sporadic cranial nerve involvement.

Swelling of the limbs occurs during the 1st year of life and may be painful. Soon thereafter, the circumference of the calvaria enlarges to 65 cm or more. Orthopedic symptoms include bending and thickening of the bones of the limbs particularly anterior bowing of the legs, and general broadening of the diaphyseal areas of the tubular bones, with loss of normal cortical outline from epiphysis to epiphysis (Fig. 7). Visual acuity may be diminished because of optic atrophy. Angioid streaks and/or macular hemorrhage have been noted. Headache is common, and hypertension has been reported in several cases. Progressive, mixed, moderately severe to severe hearing loss has

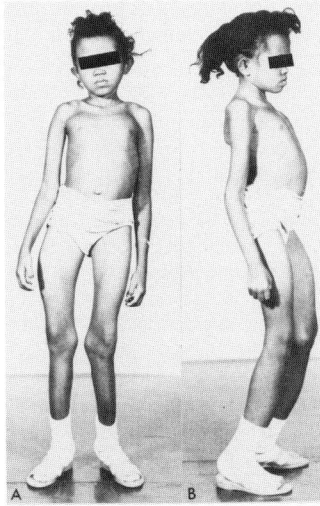

Fig. 7. Hereditary hyperphosphatasia (juvenile Paget disease): Eleven-year-old child with enlargement of skull, high forehead, wide face, and bowing of lower limbs. (From Bakwin H et al: Am J Roentgenol 91:609, 1964. with permission.)

been evident from the 4th to the 14th year of life. The ear canals are narrowed.

On radiographs, the skull changes closely resemble those seen in classic Paget disease. The long bones exhibit bending, over cylinderization, and general diaphyseal cortical widening. The bone structure is coarse. Short bones are involved to a lesser degree; the facial bones are rarely involved. Both serum acid and alkaline phosphatase levels are elevated, but calcium and phosphorus levels are normal.

REFERENCES

1. Konigsmark BW, Gorlin RJ: "Genetic and Metabolic Deafness." Philadelphia: WB Saunders, 1976.
2. Dudding BA, Gorlin RJ, Langer LO: The oto-palato-digital syndrome. Am J Dis Child 113:214–221, 1967.
3. Poznanski AK, Macpherson R, Gorlin R, Garn S, Nagy J, Gall J, Stern A, Dijkman D: The hand in the oto-palato-digital syndrom. Ann Radiol (Paris) 16:203–209, 1973.
4. Kozlowski, K, Turner G, Scougall J, Harrington J: Oto-palato-digital syndrome with severe x-ray changes in two half brothers. Pediatr Radiol 6:97–102, 1977.

5. Gorlin RJ, Poznanski AK, Hendon I: The oto-palato-digital (OPD) syndrome in females. Heterozygotic expression of an X-linked trait. Oral Surg 35:218–224, 1973.
6. Gorlin RJ, Spranger J, Koszalka MF: Genetic craniotubular bone dysplasia and hyperostoses: A critical analysis. In Bergsma D (ed): Part IV. "Skeletal Dysplasias." White Plains: The National Foundation-March of Dimes, BD:OAS V(4):79–95, 1969.
7. Beighton P, Hamersma H, Horan F: Craniometaphyseal dysplasia: Variability of expression within a large family. Clin Genet 15:252–258, 1979.
8. Cooper JC: Craniometaphyseal dysplasia. J Oral Surg 12:196–204, 1974.
9. Kietzer G, Paparella MM: Otolaryngological disorders in craniometaphyseal dysplasia. Larnygoscope 79:921–941, 1969.
10. Jackson UPU, Albright F, Drewry G, Hanelin J, Rubin MI: Metaphyseal dysplasia, epiphyseal dysplasia, diaphyseal dysplasia, and related constitutions. Arch Intern Med 94:871–884, 1954.
11. Millard DR, Maisels DO, Batstone JHF, Yates BW: Craniofacial surgery in craniometaphyseal dysplasia. Am J Surg 113:615–621, 1967.
12. Penchaszadeh VB, Gutierrez ER, Figueroa E: Autosomal recessive craniometaphyseal dysplasia. Am J Med Genet 5:43–56, 1980.
13. Halliday J: A rare case of bone dysplasia. Br J Surg 37:52–63, 1949.
14. Macpherson RI: Craniodiaphyseal dysplasia, a disease or group of diseases? J Can Assoc Radiol 25:22–23, 1974.
15. Stransky E, Mabilangan L, Lara RT: On Paget's disease with leontiasis ossea and hypothyreosis, starting in early childhood. Ann Paediatr 199:393–408, 1962.
16. Fosmoe RJ, Holm RS, Hildreth RC: Van Buchem's disease (hyperostosis corticalis generalisata familiaris). Radiology 90:771–774, 1968.
17. Gorlin RJ, Cohen MM Jr: Frontometaphyseal dysplasia. A new syndrome. Am J Dis Child 118:487–494, 1969.
18. Arenberg IK, Shambaugh GE Jr, Valvassori GE: Otolaryngologic manifestations of frontometaphyseal dysplasia. The Gorlin-Holt syndrome. Arch Otolaryngol 99:52–58, 1974.
19. Danks DM, Mayne V, Hall RK, McKinnon MC: Fronto-metaphyseal dysplasia. Am J Dis Child 123:254–258, 1972.
20. Holt JF, Thompson GR, Arenberg IK: Frontometaphyseal dysplasia. Radiol Clin North Am 10:225–243, 1972.
21. Jervis GA, Jenkins EC: Case Report #31. Syndrome Identification III(1):18–19, 1975.
22. Ullrich E, Witkowski R, Kozlowski R: Frontometaphyseal dysplasia (report of two familial cases). Aust Radiol 23:265–271, 1979.
23. Weiss L, Reynolds WA, Syzmanowski RT: Familial frontometaphyseal dysplasia—Evidence for dominant inheritance. Am J Dis Child 130:259–264, 1976.
24. Gorlin RJ, Winter RB: Frontometaphyseal dysplasia—Evidence for X-linked inheritance. Am J Med Genet 5:81–82, 1980.
25. Loria-Cortes R, Quesada-Calvo E, Cordero-Chaverri C: Osteopetrosis in children—A report of 26 cases. J Pediatr 91:43–47, 1977.
26. Myers EN, Stool S: The temporal bone in osteopetrosis. Acta Otolaryngol 89:460–469, 1969.
27. Suga F, Lindsay JR: Temporal bone histopathology of osteopetrosis. Ann Otol Rhinol Laryngol 85:15–24, 1976.
28. Gorlin RJ, Kietzer G, Wolfson J: Stapes fixation and proximal symphalangism. Z Kinderheilkd 108:12–16, 1970.

29. Spoendlin H: Congenital stapes ankylosis and fusion of carpal and tarsal bones as a dominant hereditary syndrome. Arch Otorhinolaryngol (NY) 206:173–179, 1974.
30. Vase, P, Prytz S, Pedersen PS: Congenital stapes fixation, symphalangism and syndactylia. Acta Otolaryngol 80:394–398, 1975.
31. Murakami Y: Nievergelt-Pearlman syndrome with impairment of hearing. J Bone Joint Surg 57B:367–372, 1975.
32. Maroteaux P, Bouvet JP, Briard ML: La maladie des synostosis multiples. Nouv Presse Med 1:3041–3047, 1972.
33. Herrmann J: Symphalangism and brachydactyly syndrome. Report of the *WL* symphalangism-brachydactyly syndrome. In Bergsma D (ed): "Limb Malformations." Miami: Symposia Specialists for The National Foundation-March of Dimes, BD:OAS 10(5):23–54, 1974.
34. Char F: An unusual form of brachydactyly associated with deafness. (Abstract) In Bergsma D, Lowry RB (eds): "Natural History of Birth Defects." New York: Alan R Liss for The National Foundation-March of Dimes, BD:OAS XIII(3C):228, 1977.
35. Hirsch IS: Generalized osteitis fibrosa. Radiology 13:44–84, 1929.
36. van Buchem FS, Hadders HN, Hansen JF, Woldring MG: Hyperostosis corticalis generalisata. Am J Med 33:387–396, 1962.
37. van Buchem FS: Hyperostosis corticalis generalisata. Eight new cases. Acta Med Scand 189:257–267, 1971.
38. Beighton P, Hamersma H, Durr L: The clinical features of sclerosteosis — A review of the manifestations in 25 affected individuals. Ann Intern Med 84:393–397, 1976.
39. Kniest W: Zur Abgrenzung der Dysostosis enchondralis von der Chondrodystrophie. Z Kinderheilkd 70:663–640, 1952.
40. Maroteaux P, Spranger J: La maladie de Kniest. Arch Fr Pediatr 30:735–750, 1973.
41. Kim HJ, Beratis NG, Brill P, Raab E, Hirschhorn K, Matalon R: Kniest syndrome with dominant inheritance and mucopolysacchariduria. Am J Hum Genet 27:755–764, 1975.
42. Gnamey D, Farriaux JP, Fontaine G: La maladie de Kniest. Une observation familiale. Arch Fr Pediat 33:143–151, 1976.
43. Lachman R, Rimoin DL, Hollister DW, Dorst JP, Siggers DC, McAlister W, Kaufman RL, Langer LO: The Kniest syndrome. Am J Roentgenol 123:805–814, 1975.
44. Siggers DC, Rimoin DL, Dorst JP, Doty SB, Williams BR, Hollister DW, Silberberg R, Cranley RE, Kaufman RL, McKusick VA: The Kniest disease. In Bergsma D (ed): "Skeletal Dysplasias." Miami: Symposia Specialists for The National Foundation-March of Dimes, BD:OAS X(9):193–208, 1974.
45. Bakwin H, Eiger MS: Fragile bones and macrocranium. J Pediatr 49:558–564, 1956.
46. Eyring EJ, Eisenberg E: Congenital hyperphosphatasia: A clinical, pathological, and biochemical study of two cases. J Bone Joint Surg 50A:1099–1117, 1968.
47. Marshall WC: A chronic progressive osteopathy with hyperphosphatasia. Proc R Soc Med 55:238–239, 1962.
48. Thompson RC Jr, Gaull GE, Horwitz SJ, Schenk RK: Hereditary hyperphosphatasia. Studies of three siblings. Am J Med 47:209–219, 1969.
49. Wagner JM, Solomon A: Hyperostosis corticalis infantilis (Caffey's disease). S Afr Med J 43:754–755, 1969.

Index

Albers-Schönberg disease, 78–79
Animals, deafness in, 29–30.
    See also Specific animals
Annual Survey of Hearing
    Impaired Children and
    Youth, 4–6
Audiometry, pure-tone, 47–49, 51
Auditory Brainstem Response, 47,
    52, 54, 55
Auricular malformations, 62,
    63–65
Avian middle ear, 13–15

Brainstem, and hearing loss, 47,
    48, 51. *See also* Auditory
    Brainstem Response
Branchial arch, 10–11, 19, 21,
    23–24, 63–65, 70
Branchio-oto-dysplasia, 59
Branchio-oto-renal-adysplasia,
    61–63, 70–71

Central hearing loss, 47–55
    negative evidence for, 48–49
    positive evidence for, 49–55
Children, hearing loss in, 3–7
Cortical deafness, 48, 51, 52
Craniodiaphyseal dysplasia, 76–77
Craniometaphyseal dysplasia
    dominant, 74–75
    recessive, 75–76

Deafness
    hereditary, 29–32
    nonsyndromic, 35–45

prelingual, 326
recessive, 42–43
rubella, 44–45
See also Hearing loss

Ear dysplasia-renal adysplasia
    syndrome, 59–71
    cases of, 60–63
    ear-kidney associations, 59–60
Electrocochleogram, 54, 55
Electroencephalogram, 52
Epidemiology, hearing loss
    children, 3–7
    future of, 6–7
External ear malformations, 59,
    63–71

Frontometaphyseal dysplasia, 77

Gallaudet Survey, 39–42
Galvanic Skin Response, 47, 49

Hearing loss
    age of onset, 4–5
    associated with musculoskeletal
        malformations, 73–85
    central, 47–55
    childhood, 3–7
    conductive, 79–81
    etiology of, 6, 7
    geographical distribution of,
        5–6
    hereditary, 29–32
    prevalence, 4–5
    racial distribution, 6

sensorineural, 35, 48
sex distribution, 6
See also Deafness
Hereditary
 inner ear abnormalities, 29–32
 renal adysplasia, 62–63
Heterogeneity, of deafness, 29, 36
Hyperphosphatasia, autosomal
 recessive, 84–85

Inner ear abnormalities, 29–32

Kidneys, polycystic, 62, 70
Kniest dysplasia, 83–84

Middle ear
 avian, 13–15
 developmental anatomy, 10–12
 morphogenesis, 9–26
 mouse, 12–13, 20–22
 pathogenesis of malformations, 63–71
 teratogenesis, 9–26
Mondini malformation, 61–62, 71
Mouse, middle ear, 12–13
Musculoskeletal malformation,
 73–85

National Census of the Deaf
 Population (NCDP), 4–6
National Survey, 41–42

Osteopetrosis, recessive, 78–79
Otomandibular disorders, 59
Otopalatodigital syndrome, 73
Otic capsule, 10, 11, 13–15, 20,
 25–26
Oval window (fenestra ovalis),
 10, 15–17, 20, 23

Pedigree data, segregation
 analysis of, 37–45

Renal adysplasia, *See* Ear
 dysplasia-renal adysplasia
Renal anomalies, pathogenesis
 of, 69–71
Rubella, 44–45

Sclerosteosis, 81–83
Segregation analysis, of pedigree
 data, 37–45
Speech, 47, 49–52, 55
Speech Reception Threshold, 47
Symphalangism, dominant,
 79–81
Symphalangism-brachydactyly
 syndrome, 81
Synostoses, multiple, 81

Teratogenesis, middle ear, 17–26
Triethylenemelamine, 20

Van Buchem disease, 81–83
Vitamin A, 20, 25

BOOKS PUBLISHED BY ALAN R. LISS, INC.
FOR THE NATIONAL FOUNDATION

BIRTH DEFECTS: ORIGINAL ARTICLE SERIES

1975 — Volume XI

No. 7   Morphogenesis and Malformation of Face and Brain, Daniel Bergsma and
Jan Langman, *Editors*

1976 — Volume XII

No. 1   Cancer and Genetics, Daniel Bergsma, R. Neil Schimke, Robert L. Summitt, and
David J. Harris, *Editors*

No. 3   The Eye and Inborn Errors of Metabolism, Daniel Bergsma, Anthony J. Bron, and
Edward Cotlier, *Editors*

No. 4   Developmental Disabilities: Psychologic and Social Implications, Daniel Bergsma
and Ann E. Pulver, *Editors*

No. 5   Cytogenetics, Environment and Malformation Syndromes, Daniel Bergsma and
R. Neil Schimke, *Editors*

No. 6   Growth Problems and Clinical Advances, Daniel Bergsma and R. Neil Schimke,
Editors

No. 8   Iron Metabolism and Thalassemia, Daniel Bergsma, Anthony Cerami,
Charles M. Peterson, and Joseph H. Graziano, *Editors*

1977 — Volume XIII

No. 1   Morphogenesis and Malformation of the Limb, Daniel Bergsma and
Widukind Lenz, *Editors*

No. 2   Morphogenesis and Malformation of the Genital System, Richard J. Blandau
and Daniel Bergsma, *Editors*

No. 3   Annual Review of Birth Defects, 1976, Daniel Bergsma and R. Brian Lowry,
Editors
Proceedings of the 1976 Vancouver Birth Defects Conference. Published in 4
volumes:
3A   Numerical Taxonomy of Birth Defects *and* Polygenic Disorders
3B   New Syndromes
3C   Natural History of Specific Birth Defects
3D   Embryology and Pathogenesis *and* Prenatal Diagnosis

No. 5   Urinary System Malformations in Children, Daniel Bergsma and John W. Duckett,
Editors

No. 6   Trends and Teaching in Clinical Genetics, Daniel Bergsma, Frederick Hecht,
Gerald H. Prescott, and Joan H. Marks, *Editors*

1978 — Volume XIV

No. 1   Genetic Effects on Aging, Daniel Bergsma and David E. Harrison, *Editors*

No. 2   The Molecular Basis of Cell-Cell Interaction, Richard A. Lerner and
Daniel Bergsma, *Editors*

No. 3   The Genetics of Hand Malformations, *by* Samia A. Temtamy and Victor A.
McKusick

No. 5   Neurochemical and Immunologic Components in Schizophrenia, Daniel Bergsma
and Allan L. Goldstein, *Editors*

91

No. 6   **Annual Review of Birth Defects, 1977,** Robert L Summitt and Daniel Bergsma, *Editors*
Proceedings of the 1977 Memphis Birth Defects Conference. Published in 3 volumes:
    6A   **Cell Surface Factors, Immune Deficiencies, Twin Studies**
    6B   **Recent Advances** *and* **New Syndromes**
    6C   **Sex Differentiation** *and* **Chromosomal Abnormalities**
No. 7   **Morphogenesis and Malformation of the Cardiovascular System,** Glenn C. Rosenquist and Daniel Bergsma, *Editors*

1979 — Volume XV

No. 1   **Sex Chromosome Aneuploidy: Prospective Studies on Children,** Arthur Robinson, Herbert A. Lubs, and Daniel Bergsma, *Editors*
No. 2   **Genetic Counseling: Facts, Values, and Norms,** Alexander M. Capron, Marc Lappé, Robert F. Murray, Jr., Tabitha M. Powledge, Sumner B. Twiss, and Daniel Bergsma, *Editors*
No. 3   **Recent Advances in the Developmental Biology of Central Nervous System Malformation,** Ntinos C. Myrianthopoulos and Daniel Bergsma, *Editors*
No. 4   **Continuous Transcutaneous Blood Gas Monitoring,** A. Huch, R. Huch, and J. Lucey, *Editors*
No. 5   **Annual Review of Birth Defects, 1978,** Proceedings of the 1978 San Francisco Birth Defects Conference. Published in 3 volumes:
    5A   **Diagnostic Approaches to the Malformed Fetus, Abortus, Stillborn, and Deceased Newborn,** Mitchell S. Golbus and Bryan D. Hall, *Editors*
    5B   **Penetrance and Variability in Malformation Syndromes,** James J.O'Donnell and Bryan D. Hall, *Editors*
    5C   **Risks, Communication, and Decision Making in Genetic Counseling,** Charles J. Epstein, Cynthia J.R. Curry, Seymour Packman, Sanford Sherman, and Bryan D. Hall, *Editors*
No. 6   **Dermatoglyphics — Fifty Years Later,** Wladimir Wertelecki and Chris C. Plato, *Editors*
No. 7   **Newborn Behavioral Organization: Nursing Research and Implications,** Gene Cranston Anderson and Beverly Raff, *Editors*
No. 8   **Developmental Aspects of Craniofacial Dysmorphology,** Michael Melnick and Ronald Jorgenson, *Editors*
No. 9   **External Ear Malformations: Epidemiology, Genetics, and Natural History,** *by* Michael Melnick and Ntinos C. Myrianthopoulos